OUT ABOUT

A TRAVEL AND TRANSPORT GUIDE

CW01023647

*Developed for publication
by Richard Armitage and
John Taylor of the
Community Transport
Association.*

AGE *Concern*

NATIONAL EXPRESS »
CALEDONIAN EXPRESS »

© 1990
Age Concern England
1268 London Road
London SW16 4ER

Editor   Eddie Dyja
Design   Eugenie Dodd
Production   Joyce O'Shaughnessy
Illustrations   Sal Shuel
Printed by Grosvenor Press, Portsmouth

British Library Cataloguing in Publication Data
Out and About: a travel and transport guide.
   I. Transport services for old persons
   I. Armitage. Richard   II. Taylor, John *1952 Apr. 25.*
   III. Age Congern England.
   388.0420846

ISBN 0 86242 092 X

The cover illustration is reproduced by kind permission of the
London Transport Museum.

Age Concern England would like to acknowledge the generous
financial sponsorship provided by National Express to allow
this book to reach a wider audience.

Contents

Contents

PART 3

Further information 149

Foreword

The last few years have seen more and more people travelling further and further afield; however, this new found freedom has increased the concerns faced by older people when travelling.

How many of these concerns are an inevitable result of the pace of modern life is debatable. What is certain is that more people than ever before want to be able to keep their mobility and independence. Consequently, transport operators recognise the importance of this group of customers and are striving to make travel as easy and as convenient as possible. They now realise that, whether a journey is to the local shops or the other side of the world, people need help, information and reassurance.

I am delighted therefore, to have assisted Age Concern in their Golden Jubilee year with the production of this guide giving details on getting 'out and about'.

As the leading operator of express coach services in Great Britain, National Express and Caledonian Express are making a special effort to look after the needs of older passengers, many of whom come back to us time after time.

New coaches, fitted with reclining seats, curtains, toilets, a front step that can be lowered to the ground and carrying a hostess or steward, are entering service throughout the country. Discounts on fares of around 30 per cent are available to anyone aged 60 and over and special assistance is available at many coach stations to make your journey as comfortable and as enjoyable as possible.

Details of how coach travel, along with many other forms of public and private transport, is making it easier to get out and about, will be found in this excellent guide.

We look forward to being of service to you in the future.

Bernard Davis
Marketing Director, National Express

About the Authors

Richard Armitage
Editor of *Community Transport Magazine*, previously General Secretary of the Community Transport Association (1984-90).

Dr. Caroline Cahm
Secretary of 'Buswatch', the passengers' national monitoring project; Chairman of the National Federation of Bus Users.

Michael Dearing
Secretary of the National Federation of Bus Users since 1985; member of the Consumer Congress Transport Working Party.

Brian Howard
Development Officer for TRIPSCOPE, a telephone-based travel and transport information service for elderly and disabled people.

Graham Lightfoot
Obtained Transport Management and Planning Degree in 1976; since then has been organising, researching and writing about community transport.

Barbara Preston
Principal lecturer, Manchester Polytechnic, now retired; Vice-President of the Pedestrians Association.

Michelle Le Prevost
Recently completed six years as Age Concern Hampshire's Voluntary Transport Development Officer.

Paul Salveson
Just spent three years as Transport Development Worker with Greater Manchester Council of Voluntary Service; previously, six years with British Rail.

John Taylor
Transport consultant specialising in community and voluntary transport; Technical and Legal Adviser to the Community Transport Association.

Ian Yearsley
Freelance journalist specialising in public transport matters; previous editorial appointments include *Railway Gazette International, Motor Transport,* and *Urban Transport International.*

Preface

This guide provides a handy source of information on travel, which lets you plan a journey from the comfort of your own armchair. It is a single, comprehensive starting point for making a successful trip. Throughout the guide, we emphasise that getting older can increase your travel opportunities. The message is straightforward and appealing:

YOU CAN GET THERE!

Out and About is divided into three parts: in the first, we cover how to plan your travel, to make it as pleasant as possible; in the second, we look at the many different ways you can travel, to help you choose the right way to go; and at the end, we provide a list of useful addresses.

Richard Armitage and John Taylor

Acknowledgements

Thanks to Caroline Freedman for her thorough research work.

Thanks also to Age Concern England staff for continuous help and support – in particular, Ben Plowden, Evelyn McEwen, David Moncrieff, Margaret McLellan and Vinnette Marshall.

Introduction

Travel is good for you. It broadens the mind, but it also plays an important part in leading a healthy and active life. Being able to get about, whether it is to the local shops, a neighbouring town or the other side of the world, is something that most people take for granted.

Later life presents a perfect opportunity to travel, as work and family responsibilities give way to more free time. Not everyone wants to go round the world, but even the most local trip can be worthwhile and interesting.

However, as people get older, their ability to get about may become more limited. This can be for any number of reasons. They may be financially constrained. They may become physically less able to get about. They may lack the confidence or inclination to make the journeys they made formerly. A great many of these obstacles can be overcome if the right information is available.

Knowing how to get from A to B affordably and comfortably is the first step in any journey. How do I find out about the bus services to the new supermarket? Is there a coach or train direct to my daughter's home town? Will there be someone to help me with my luggage? Are there any reduced fares for people over 60?

Having this information, or knowing where to look for it, gives people greatly enhanced opportunities for travel, and the enjoyment and fulfillment that goes with it. Not having this information before setting off can make even the most simple journey tiring, worrying and unnecessarily expensive.

Many people are confident and experienced travellers. For them, *Out and About* will be a valuable source of information for new trips or old trips being taken again. Some people, however, may not be so confident, or may have resources that only allow for an occasional trip.

Whatever the case, *Out and About* contains information about all sorts of travel possibilities in a clear and concise way. It gives details on all the main ways of travelling. Comparisons are made between different ways of making the same journey, to help identify the kind of 'false economies' that can arise if a cheap but not so cheerful option is chosen. In particular, the book is designed to help in the all important planning of a journey – who to ask, what to ask them, what to take, when to leave and when to arrive.

In addition, the book contains an invaluable selection of contact addresses and telephone numbers for organisations that may come in useful before or during a trip.

Of course, no amount of information will be able to overcome some obstacles. There is still a long way to go before everybody can go out and about where and when they choose. Elderly people can face a number of difficulties when it comes to maintaining mobility. For example, they are discriminated against in the area of disability benefits. Mobility Allowance is a benefit providing financial help towards transport costs, but people are disqualified from receiving Mobility Allowance if they become disabled after the age of 65. The costs of being disabled do not necessarily fall with age, and Age Concern believes that this discrimination is unjustifiable and should be ended.

Overall, transport and land-use policy in this country severely discriminates against people without access to a car, and this includes a majority of elderly people. Only 40 per cent of households in which there is at least one older person have a car. This falls to 12 per cent of households made up of a single older person, compared with 72 per cent of households containing no older people. In recent years, we have seen an ever-increasing concentration of many public and private services, including huge out-of-town shopping centres, health services and leisure facilities. This has been accompanied by a corresponding decline in local facilities that can be reached on foot and by public transport. These developments are fine for people with access to a car, but can severely diminish the quality of life of many elderly people dependent on walking and local buses. We believe that transport and planning policies should take into account the needs of everybody, not just car owners, so that those without cars are not denied access to their chosen activities. However, while we should not forget these difficulties, this book will be a useful guide for people who want to explore different travel possibilities at home before making a journey, and may make trips possible that appear impossible at first sight. Its basic message is, get up and go!

Sally Greengross
Director, Age Concern England

Note

Throughout this book we have cited examples of prices which were correct when the book was being written. The actual prices are likely to change but they are still included so that you can gauge the differences.

PART

You can get there *Being able to get out and about as much as possible is important for a healthy and independent life. Research has shown that keeping active can help people stay mentally and physically alert.*

Older people have far more leisure time than in the past. Commercial transport operators and holiday firms recognise you as part of a growing market which they are keen to serve.

Retirement can open up wonderful opportunities to do all the things and visit all the people and places that you have never had time for.

In order to travel well, you will need to plan your journey and with the right information you can have an enjoyable time.

PLANNING

Richard Armitage

Importance of planning

Planning is the first stage of your journey. It enables you to have a good trip, because you know all the costs, you have checked the connections, your paperwork is in order and you have the facts at your finger-tips.

In this chapter, you will find a series of planning tips and hints. Taken together, they form the basis for a detailed travel plan for even the longest and most complex journey.

All journeys involve some degree of planning, and the longer they are, the more is needed. Planning minimises the risks of problems cropping up during the journey. But it also makes sure you find the best way of making the trip in the first place.

Choosing the right way to go

Different ways of travelling will be appropriate for different journeys. Each method of travelling will have different costs and considerations, such as the time taken to complete the journey, the comfort and the convenience.

There are plenty of options to choose from:

- walking vs cycling
- local bus vs taxi
- car vs taxi/bus/cycling/train/coach/air/walking
- air vs train
- train vs coach

Opposite are two examples which compare various travelling options with cost, time, comfort, convenience and pleasure.

EXAMPLE ■
Manchester – Edinburgh *Centre-to-centre*

MONEY *Lowest return fare*
Air	*£85 inc. buses between airport and city centre*
Train	*£15.20 with a Senior Railcard*
Coach	*£11.00*
Car	**Mileage £51.60** *430 miles at 12 pence per mile – marginal costs only*

TIME *Each way*
Air	*Flight takes 65 minutes; with bus rides, a total of 2 hours*
Train	*Four hours*
Coach	*Six hours*
Car	*Five to Six hours assuming a meal stop*

COMFORT
Air	*May find it noisy during flight, lap belt compulsory*
Train	*Good*
Coach	*More cramped than trains, but seats comfortable*
Car	*Depends on your car*

CONVENIENCE
Air	*Free newspapers, snack and light refreshments in-flight; fastest journey time*
Train	*Centre-to-centre; on-board refreshments; less tiring than driving*
Coach	*Centre-to-centre; stops once at motorway service station; cheapest option*
Car	*You can take the kitchen sink; door-to-door, but allow time and money for parking in the city centres*

PLEASURE FACTORS
Air	*Spectacular views (eg Firth of Forth) if the weather's fine*
Train	*You can stretch your legs during the journey*
Coach	*You can get some fresh air at motorway service station stop*
Car	*You can take the scenic route*

EXAMPLE 2

Manchester – Belfast *Centre-to-centre*

MONEY *Lowest return fare*

Air	**£103** *inc buses between airport and city centre*
Train/Ferry	**£46.75** *plus fares in Liverpool and Belfast*
Coach/Ferry	**£50.50**
Car/Ferry	**£143** *car with driver only or*
	£181 *car and up to four people;*
	Mileage £10.20 *85 miles at 12 pence per mile – marginal costs only*

TIME *Each way*

Air	*Flight takes 60 minutes; with bus rides, no more than two hours*
Train/Ferry	*About 12 hours (nine hours on the ferry)*
Coach/Ferry	*17 hours (inc. travelling overnight)*
Car/Ferry	*About 12 hours (nine hours on the ferry)*

COMFORT, CONVENIENCE AND PLEASURE FACTORS	*Broadly similar to those in Example 1 (above). However, note that the Ferry crossing could be unpleasant if the sea is rough. The only scenic route available for the motorist is if you go via Stranraer; however this adds at least 400 miles to the round trip, and the ferry to Larne is more expensive.*

In both these examples, other 'costs' (not all of them financial) need to be taken into account before you make your mind up.

Food is a consideration on most long trips. Taking Example 1, if you are going to 'eat out', would you prefer an Edinburgh restaurant, a British Rail buffet or a motorway service station?

In Example 2, let us say that your final destination was London-derry: air travel is the only option which would allow you to do the trip comfortably in a day; both the train and the car would arrive about 10.30 pm, so you would have the additional cost of bed and breakfast; the coach arrives at 10.30 am, but unless you were able to sleep well on the coach and ferry, it is unlikely travelling even further would give you much pleasure.

The timing of a trip can be crucial: in large towns and cities, you need to take into account the morning and evening peak travel period during weekdays; be aware of public holidays, when some services you require may be unavailable or the major roads may be crowded; and when and where you would like to eat, or stay overnight.

Making a booking

It is possible to book trips and holidays and order tickets by telephone with ease, especially if you are paying with a credit card. But whether you are making the booking in person or over the phone, planning beforehand will save you time and money.

Always enquire when booking your travel whether the company can give you special rates; eg for being over 60, or whether they are doing any special deals; eg two adults travel at the same price during October.

CASE HISTORY

In March, Alice and John decide they are going to do something different for their holiday. They go to their local travel agent for information on farmhouse holidays in France. They spend a few weeks looking through the brochures. They want to go at the end of May, because they do not want the weather to be too hot. In April, they have made up their mind, but the travel agent says: "Sorry, but they're already full up".

This example shows the importance of booking in good time so your plans will not be upset. You can check out availability and many other questions at your local travel agent. Most travel agents will be pleased to put together a 'package' for you.

Tickets for standard trips can also be bought in advance directly from the operator (British Rail, National Express, airlines, ferry companies and so on). It is worth reserving a seat at any time of year (see Checklist, on page 19); but it is essential during high season and public holidays.

Making the connections

Before you set off, check the connections. Allow plenty of time to transfer yourself and any luggage between arrival and departure. Getting connections wrong is not only a frustrating business, but a costly one: a big delay will mean a meal has to be bought as well. You may even find that an earlier or later service goes straight through, thus avoiding having to change at all. As a rule, only connect with a final service of the day if it is completely unavoidable. A missed connection would mean an unplanned overnight stay in a hotel or guest house. However, every cloud has a silver lining: if it is late and a local hotel is your only option, do not forget to discuss the price with them. Your negotiating position is not as weak as you might think; to the hotel, you are filling an extra bed they had not managed to sell.

Making your exit

Do you know when to get off? Stopping at the right point in a journey requires just as much thinking ahead as starting it:

Look up your exit's junction number before you set off up the motorway.

Make sure the bus (or train) is stopping where you want it to and is not a through service that by-passes your destination.

If you think you might fall asleep on the way ask another passenger to nudge you awake when your stop is approaching.

Insurance

The perfect insurance policy is one that covers you for any eventuality, including civil war and earthquakes. In the real world, this policy has yet to be written. However, these days you can get fairly close. You can always get detailed advice from your registered insurance broker or accredited insurance agent. Never travel abroad without insurance, especially medical and accident cover.

CHECKLIST: MAKING A BOOKING

Journey:
- From: . . . To: . . . Via: . . .

How much do I want to spend?
- On travel?
- When I get there?

Dates and times of travel:
- Out: . . .   Return: . . .
- Times: . . .   Times: . . .
- Check-in times (coaches, ferries, airlines)

During the journey:
- Toilet and wash-room facilities?
- Food?
- Seat reservation:
  Smoking or non-smoking?
  Rear or forward-facing?
  Aisle or window?
  With a companion – seated together or opposite each other?
  Recliner/cabin? (Ferry)

Accommodation required?
- Bed and breakfast?
- Full board or half board?
- Dates?
- Meals required?

Taxi or bus required?

Currency required?
- Travellers' cheques required?
- Car hire at the other end?

Someone to meet me when I arrive?

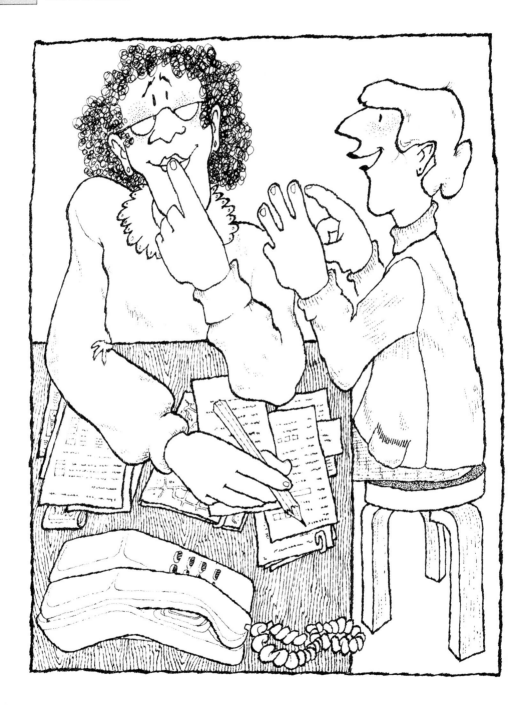

You should first of all check the small print of your house insurance policy. This may provide cover for your luggage and its contents when you are away from home. Find out whether important valuables, such as your camera and jewellery, are excluded or cash limited. You may find it economical to extend your house cover rather than take out a fresh policy.

Your house policy should also have a section on money, including credit cards. In many instances, this should be more than sufficient cover for your travelling needs.

For peace of mind, you can get one-off travel insurance, especially if you are going abroad. This will offer a package of benefits:

- personal accident cover
- medical expenses cover, including hospital benefits
- cancellation, curtailment and travel delay cover
- baggage cover
- money cover
- personal liability cover.

The amount you pay will be related to where in the world you are going, and how long you will be away. Read the small print carefully, as the policies offered vary considerably in the benefits they provide. For example, although the baggage cover may be for £1,000, it may have a maximum pay-out of £100 for any single item lost or stolen.

If you are paying for your travel by credit card, check out whether they provide some form of automatic travel insurance cover.

Paperwork

You can write off potential travel problems by getting all the paperwork sorted out well in advance, and then all you have to do is keep a check that it is up-to-date. In particular, do not get caught out trying to get a passport or visa at the last minute: you could end up having to queue for hours outside the issuing office.

CHECKLIST: DOCUMENTS

To be carried at all times:

- special medical requirements or medic alert pendant
- donor card
- emergency: please contact . . . (phone and address of next-of-kin, friend and so on) . . .
- tickets
- booking confirmation

Travelling in Britain:

- bus pass
- railcard
- Disabled Person's Railcard

Travelling abroad: (see section on Going Abroad page 96)

- passport
- visa(s)
- inoculation certificate(s)
- insurance cover information
- health: Form E111

Travelling in your own car: (see section on Cars page 58)

- driving licence
- copy of Insurance Certificate
- copy of MoT Certificate
- motoring organisation membership card
- abroad – Green Card
- abroad – International Driving Licence

Another set of 'documents' that may come in handy: five minutes spent in a photo booth will provide you with four ready-to-use passport-size recent pictures of yourself. You need one for your bus pass, for museum passes, for your weekly pass, most ski-lifts now require one, and so on.

Watching your cash

Banks, building societies, travel agents, hoteliers and the police never tire of warning you to take care with your money. Here, for the record, is another appeal to watch your cash when you are on the move.

The first rule is don't carry lots of cash with you. Only carry as much as you are going to spend that day (or weekend), with perhaps a little extra for unexpected expense.

The second rule is to make it very difficult for someone to take your cash without your knowledge; this is especially hard when it is warm and you are wearing fewer clothes (eg swimming). A wallet should never be kept in a back trouser pocket; a purse in an open handbag or shopping trolley is inviting trouble. Bags that zip shut and have straps that can go over the opposite shoulder are harder to snatch. Other options include wearing a money belt or pouch, or attaching a chain from your belt or coat to the wallet or purse.

The third rule is to carry your money in other forms. Even if it is stolen, you can make it difficult or impossible for the thief to become rich. Credit cards, travellers' cheques, standard cheque books, Giro books (cashable at the Post Office), and building society account books are all designed to make thieving less rewarding. Do not keep your credit cards with your cheque book; do keep a separate list of your account and card numbers back at the hotel (with a copy back home) with the emergency telephone numbers to ring in case of theft or loss.

Should the worst occur, and you have to choose between parting with your money or being attacked, decide in advance to hand over your money.

Clothing sense

Sensible clothing and appropriate footwear are good travelling companions. Modern, good quality waterproofs come in a range of colours and styles, thanks to the new materials (such as Goretex).

The initial outlay is not cheap, but should last you many years. Look out for the anoraks and coats that have detachable quilted inners, to keep you warm in winter.

But it is not all about wet, windy or cold weather. Your aim must be to travel in comfort, matching what you wear to the conditions. If it is in the eighties, a good sun hat and lightweight cottons are essential to keep you cool.

You may be travelling – on a long flight for example – in both cool and warm conditions. The only answer is to take several layers and be prepared to adjust as the trip unfolds. Take a small bag or rucksack to keep the spare clothes in.

If you are walking beside roads, BE SEEN. The driver may not see you if you are wearing a dark grey overcoat for instance.

Luggage

Whether you are merely walking to the Post Office or going on a round-the-world whirl, make 'travel light and easy' your motto.

But first, a word about hand-held bags. The problem with these is that you have to hold them at all times. They are also easily snatched by a thief. So, why not carry your essentials on your back? Specialist travel shops, such as those run by the Youth Hostels Association (see p 150) now have a wide range of small backpacks and rucksacks: they are lightweight, strong, as colourful as you wish and exceedingly comfortable to wear. With the items you need for the day on your back, you leave both hands free.

If you still want to use a hand-held bag, get one with a full length, detachable shoulder strap, preferably with a padded wider section where it goes across your shoulder. You should wear the strap diagonally across your shoulder and around your body.

You should try to put all other items on wheels. You can either buy suitcases with wheels already attached, or you can buy lightweight mini-trolleys, which fold away and stow in your suitcase itself or in another bag.

When packing for a journey, split the task into two: there are those essential items you will need during the trip, and the things you want when you have arrived.

Essential items to have on hand during a journey include:

- money and paperwork
- food and drink
- reading matter
- camera
- medicines

As a rule, the more experienced the traveller, the less he or she carries about with them. If you are going somewhere interesting, it would be far more fun to buy clothes and so on when you get there – it may also be cheaper than getting them at home.

Look after yourself

It is surprising how hungry you can get when travelling, so make sure you always carry a little food to keep you going. This is especially important if you get delayed en route. A cheese sandwich, a slice of fruitcake, crisps, fresh fruit, and biscuits are all easy to carry and consume whilst you are in transit.

It is just as important to avoid getting thirsty. Dehydration can quickly make you tired, and will lessen your enjoyment of the trip. Why not carry a flask of tea, coffee, juice or mineral water? Or try one of the individual portion drinks.

Peace of mind

Whilst you are away, you do not want to spend the whole time fretting about whether you remembered to shut the bathroom window. Take the precaution of leaving a key with a trusted neighbour or friend; ask them to go round and check your home every few days; you can return the favour when they go away.

THINGS TO DO WHEN YOU ARE GOING AWAY

- leave your holiday address and insurance details with a relative or friend
- board your pets
- ask someone to look after any indoor plants
- deposit valuables and important papers with your bank
- cancel milk, newspapers and any other daily or weekly deliveries
- empty and defrost the fridge; if you have a freezer, remind your friend to check it is working properly
- wherever possible, switch off appliances, pull electric plugs out of sockets; if practical, switch off gas, electric, water and central heating
- leave a spare key with someone or somewhere safe
- if you are going to be away for some time, tell the police

If you do not have anyone you feel you can rely on, why not call in at your local Age Concern Group and see if they will find a trusted volunteer to help you out?

Frailty and disability

It is often suggested that the biggest handicap faced by a disabled person is other people. Travel and passenger transport operators are at last beginning to realise the importance of staff training in 'disability awareness', and 'customer care'. Many people with disabilities dream of the day when they can go on a trip without having to make any special arrangements. However, until then, there are a few points worth noting.

If you have 'special needs', it is best to mention them when you are making your booking, rather than waiting until you arrive. Never apologise for making demands on the services you are wanting to use; you are the paying customer, after all. In truth, many transport operators should be apologising to you for the generally poor standard of access to their services.

If you need someone to accompany you on your journey, whether this is a friend or carer, do not be afraid to ask whether there are concessions.

If your particular condition makes predicting your 'off' days especially tricky, insist that there will be no difficulties should you have to cancel at the last minute (see also Insurance, this section on page 18).

If you are hard of hearing or deaf, it is worth carrying a writing pad and pen, to make communication easier when you are travelling.

FURTHER READING

- *Holidays in the British Isles 1990: A Guide for Disabled People,* published by RADAR, price £4.50 inc. p & p. Available from branches of WH Smith, price £3.00.

- *Holiday Factsheets* published by RADAR, set of 13, price 50p each, inc. p&p.

- *Life in the Sun* by Nancy Tuft, published by Age Concern England, price £6.95.

ACCESS
John Taylor

It is one thing to choose a mountaineering holiday, but if you have to do the same sort of exercise just to get into your hotel bedroom, the fun of an outing could be spoilt. It is far better to have set off knowing that the hotel has lifts.

Barrier-free zones

The question of barrier-free buildings and other amenities has been tackled by disablement groups under the heading 'Access'. Although mainly concentrating on the needs of wheelchair users, much of the information available is of benefit to those beginning to find walking strenuous, or whose sight or hearing is not as acute as it used to be.

Access guides

On the basis that 'forewarned is forearmed', most major towns and cities (eg Cardiff) have Access Guides. These list local shops, offices, theatres, restaurants and other amenities, and offer information about how easy their facilities are to use. The kind of items covered are:

- ramps
- the number of steps
- induction loops, for use with a 'T'-switch on a hearing aid
- ground floor toilets
- lifts
- door widths (for people in wheelchairs)
- reserved parking, close by

These can make the difference between a successful journey and an inconvenient one.

Information

The Royal Association for Disability and Rehabilitation (RADAR) (see p 150) acts as a central supply point for these access guides, and also has guides covering the Channel Ports, Paris, and Israel.

Many other organisations publish booklets indicating accessibility to their facilities. A leaflet from the Royal Society for the Protection of Birds (see p 150), for example, indicates accessibility to its various hides and reserves across the country. One problem has been the lack of any objective standards when it comes to grading access, with the international wheelchair symbol often being used inappropriately. The English Tourist Board (see p 150) has recently published a report suggesting they will take the lead to improve this. In addition, they have called for every company involved in the tourist industry to have a written statement outlining its commitment to 'Tourism for All'.

Ring before you go

If there is a particular place you need to know about, then telephone in advance. Not only may you be surprised to find that something quite unlikely is, in fact, easy to get into, but this may also stimulate an offer of assistance. This is particularly true of airports, and coach and rail stations. Before you telephone, make a note of the specific things you need to know.

CHECKLIST: TEN CONSIDERATIONS

1 How far will I need to walk from . . . (nearest public transport point, or car park) . . .?

2 Is it uphill?

3 Are there any steps? If so how many?

4 Are there lifts or escalators available?

5 Are there any facilities for people who are hard of hearing or partially sighted?

6 Are there places to sit down and take a rest? If outdoors, are these sheltered?

7 How long will it take me to get round?

8 Where is the nearest toilet? Is it easily accessible?

9 Where will I be able to get a cup of tea and a snack?

10 Is there a member of staff who can assist me if I need help?

Insist on getting the detailed information you require. Do not accept a general reassurance that the location is suitable – the person at the other end of the telephone is unlikely to be an expert in this field. You are the expert on this occasion.

Accommodation

If you need help in choosing an accessible hotel, or a holiday, then the Holiday Care Service (see p 150) will assist you. This organisation provides free information, and holds details of suitable hotels and self-catering accommodation around the country, and abroad.

Toilets

A particular problem for some people is whether there will be a toilet, and whether they will be able to use it. Often public conveniences are kept locked because of vandalism. However, many toilets for disabled people, generally unisex and designed with extra space, handrails and fittings at convenient heights, have a lock which accepts the a special key available through the National Key Scheme. This key can be obtained from participating local authorities for those people who need to use adapted toilets. The key is also available, at a small charge, from RADAR (see p 150) along with a list of all the relevant toilets.

Let them know

If you can see how access can be improved, don't be shy: tell the manager or owner of the facility. They will generally welcome constructive criticism. Architects, planners and designers do not always know what is required by older people.

FURTHER READING

- *AA Guide for the Disabled Traveller 1990,* published by AA – lists accommodation throughout the UK as well as information about public conveniences, picnic sites and motorway service areas, price £3.50 from AA centres or credit card orders/orders by post to AA Publications Centre, free to members.

- *AA The World Wheelchair Traveller,* published by AA – information on travelling by road, rail, sea and air in the UK and abroad, also customs, currency and medical matters, price £3.95 from AA centre and booksellers.

- *Facilities for Disabled and Visually Handicapped Visitors,* published by The National Trust – a free guide to National Trust properties in England and Wales. The National Trust is making particular efforts in this field, and plans to provide electric-powered golf buggies at houses or gardens where access is steep or difficult. There is a similar guide for Scotland (National Trust for Scotland).

- *Gardens of England and Wales:* the National Garden Scheme – annual guide to over 220 gardens, price £1.50 from bookshops.

- *Spectators Access Guide for Disabled People,* published by RADAR – a guide to facilities and access at sporting venues in England and Wales, price £3.00 inc. p & p.

MONEY

John Taylor

The old saying 'Time is money' is particularly true when considering people who have retired. For whilst the disposable income of pensioners is less than that of people in work, the amount of time they have available enables them to seek out bargains, and travel off-peak at reduced rates, thus converting time into money.

It is sometimes assumed that older people travel less than the rest of the population, because they are no longer at work, nor in full-time education. However, research has shown * that – once you have extracted travel to work or school from the figures – as far as shopping, holidays or day trips are concerned, people over 60 travel only a little less than the rest of the population.

All this has to be paid for, and transport costs make up between 4 per cent and 8 per cent of the average household budget of the over-60s. Obviously, significant numbers of older people do restrict their travel on financial grounds, but the figures show that very many are, in fact, getting out and about. A key reason for this is that money is not everything when it comes to travelling.

* The National Travel Survey: 1985/1986 Report – Part 1, An Analysis of Personal Travel.

Economics of travel

Your aim should be to balance the cost of travel against comfort, convenience, and the pleasure it brings you. As Examples 1 and 2 demonstrated (see pp 15-16), it is not always obvious which method of travelling is going to be the best.

The car and the train both take you city centre to city centre (Example 1), but the £35+ that you save going by train could pay for at least one day's car hire (or several taxi rides) when you get there.

The train may be cheaper than the airline (Example 2: train and ferry

£46.75, air £103), but it takes far longer to get there, so you have to buy meals during the trip and arrive just in time to go to bed.

Where appropriate you will find cost comparisons throughout this guide, which will help you make the right decision, balancing your budget with your expectations about the journey.

Off-peak travel

Bus, train, plane and holiday operators all have to deal with the problem of what they do with their services outside the peak times and seasons. The most common solution is to tempt extra passengers by offering bargain rate off-peak travel. So quite apart from any concessions which are specifically available to older people, it will be cheaper not to travel during the rush hour, or high summer. British Rail 'saver' fares are a classic case in point, with the off-peak fare for a journey less than one-third the full fare. Apart from the money, you will find it far less of a rush.

Concessions

The different types of concessionary fares for older people are described in detail in the relevant sections later on in this book. It is important to keep aware of the regular concessions and get hold of your railcard, bus pass, or whatever in good time. Also keep an eye open for particular bargains. For example, for one month every year, generally November, British Rail have been offering saver tickets (to any destination, at a very reduced rate) to Senior Railcard holders. This is when you should make those spontaneous visits to friends who live on the other side of the country.

Winter in the sun

One area where older people have made use of cheap off-peak rates is in wintering abroad, particularly in Spain. The hotels and staff are there, and it is worthwhile for the owners to keep them open at very low prices, just to cover the overhead costs. Some people take a three month holiday in the Mediterranean each year over

Christmas. The weather is generally better, and lots of friendships can be made. Travel companies now offer deals which can often work out as cheap as staying at home.

The main savings are on:

- heating bills
- food (on an inclusive holiday)
- telephone bills
- car expenses
- television rental
- general household expenses

Government help

There are some direct cash benefits available from the Government to help with transport costs. Information about these benefits, and the leaflets mentioned below, are available from your nearest Social Security Office, Citizens Advice Bureau, or Age Concern group. If you just want to get hold of a leaflet, you can write to the local or head office of the Department of Social Security or telephone Freephone 0800 666555.

Mobility Allowance is a weekly cash benefit paid to severely disabled people who are unable to walk or have severe difficulty in walking. It is not taxable and not taken into account when other benefits are being calculated. You can claim Mobility Allowance if you are under 66. If you are 65, you must be able to show that you were in a position to qualify immediately before your 65th birthday. Providing you satisfy the requirements, Mobility Allowance will continue to be paid until you reach 80. People in receipt of Mobility Allowance may be exempt from paying the Road Fund Licence on their car. Information about Mobility Allowance can be found in social security leaflet NI211: *Mobility Allowance*. The rules are currently being reviewed, so check whether there have been any changes introduced.

War Pensioners Mobility Supplement is a cash benefit intended to help war pensioners who have serious problems in walking due to their pensioned disablement which must be assessed at 20 per cent or more. It cannot be claimed at the same time as Mobility Allowance, but unlike Mobility Allowance, there are no age limitations. Further information is available in social security leaflet MPL 153: *Guide for the War Disabled.*

There is a scheme for reimbursing the money which people with low incomes have to spend on getting to hospital (see Hospital, on page 104).

Travel agencies and holiday firms

Make sure the travel agent or tour operator you are using is a member of the Association of British Travel Agents (ABTA) (see p 151), for your own peace of mind. ABTA run a system of bonds, which ensures that if one of their members' firms closes down, you will either be guaranteed your original booking or you will get your money back.

Cars *see section on Cars page 58*

The chances are that a car is one of the largest purchases you will ever make, after your own home. Therefore if you are considering whether to buy one, or to continue running one, it is important you make a good choice, for the right reasons.

Cost will be a significant factor, so consider whether you will need a car on a regular basis. Cars can be expensive to run and, if your capital is important to you, lose their value quickly. If you only use it for weekend trips or when friends and relatives come to visit, hiring for a short period could be a cheaper alternative (£120 – £200 per week, plus fuel).

However, many older people living in towns have found that a car is no longer necessary. For the money they save in fuel, insurance, and so on, together with interest on the money they get from selling their existing car, they can buy a lot of taxi, bus and train journeys. They start to treat taxis as necessary public transport, rather than a luxury mode of travel.

EXAMPLE 3

Assuming a car worth £5,000 on purchase, doing 3,000 miles a year, (just under 60 miles a week) for five years. At the end of the five year period, the car is worth £1,500.

ANNUAL FIXED COSTS WOULD BE

Depreciation	£700
Insurance	£110
Tax	£100
Parking	£40
Cleaning	£20
Total	**£970**

RUNNING COSTS WOULD BE

Petrol	6.3 *pence per mile*
Tyres	0.7
Repairs, servicing, etc.	5.0
Total	**12.0** *pence per mile*

THE WEEKLY COST WOULD THUS BE

Depreciation	£13.46
Other fixed costs	£5.19
Running costs	£6.92
Total	**£25.57**

If instead of running the car, the £5,000 is invested to give a 12 per cent return, a saving will be made over the five year period. Allowing for 25 per cent tax to be paid on the £600 annual interest, this would still give a weekly income of £8.65 to add to the £12.11 already budgeted for the car's 'other fixed costs' and 'running costs'. This gives a total of £20.76 per week available for expenditure on transport which would otherwise have been done by car. This could certainly be used to buy bus and taxi journeys amounting to 60 miles each week:

Ten × 4 mile bus journeys at 25p (half fare) = £2.50
Five × 4 mile taxi journeys at £3.50 = £17.50

It would allow you to travel from Manchester to Birmingham and back four times a week (by coach, at £5.50 return).

Some people do not take depreciation into account (they do not put money aside into a 'sinking fund'), so the above figures can be expressed another way, by making a comparison between two couples, the Carrs and the Busseys, both of whom start off with £5,000.

CASE HISTORY

The Carrs buy a car with their own money. They then spend £12.11 per week in order to drive 60 miles a week. At the end of five years, they have an asset worth £1,500.

The Busseys invest their money. This gives them £8.65 per week income from the interest. They then spend £20.76 per week in order to cover 60 miles on public transport. At the end of five years, they have investments of £5,000.

On the other hand, it should be stressed that the Carrs take the view that they have accumulated capital during their working life precisely so that they can spend it during their retirement. They do not see retirement as a time to continue saving, so they plan to run down their capital over this period, and enjoy themselves whilst they are doing it.

KEEPING YOUR TRAVEL BUDGET LOW

Here are ten suggestions for saving money on travel:

1 Develop a network of friends and relatives with whom you can go and stay in return for them coming to see you. This sort of exchange, designed to save accommodation costs, obviously requires a certain amount of sensitivity to ensure that you are really welcome. Provided the arrangements are clear at the start, it should be a satisfying way to see other parts of this country and abroad, and have the fun of showing other people around all your local places of interest.

2 Get to know the tourist offices in the area you are visiting – they are a source of free maps, leaflets and information about things to do, and where to eat at a reasonable price.

3 Get a copy of *Britain for Free* from the Automobile Association (see p 150). This book lists all the museums, archaeological sites and other places of interest where no entry charge is made.

4 Guest houses, bed and breakfast, and the Youth Hostels Association (see p 150 – older people are welcome) offer substantially cheaper accommodation than hotels. Spend the money you save on having a big meal at lunch (set menus, fixed prices, excellent value), rather than at night.

5 Always ask if there are discounts available for older people. Carry some sort of proof of age with you, such as a senior citizen bus pass.

6 Organisers of outings of a certain size will generally get to travel free. So why not get together a group of friends and hire a coach for the day, or buy a group ticket?

7 Make friends with your travel agent, and be prepared to travel at short notice. They may be able to organise very cheap last minute trips for you.

8 Take care with taxis, particularly from airports. Make sure that you know how the fare is going to be calculated before you get in the vehicle.

9 If the trip or holiday wasn't satisfactory, write to the company involved saying so, and ask for some or all of your money back. Keep a copy of this letter. If the worst comes to the worst, there are codes of practice for travel agents and tour operators, and you can have any dispute adjudicated on independently.

10 Take your own packed lunch, and a flask – it may be tastier, as well as cheaper, than much of the food available at coach and rail stations.

SUMMARY
Richard Armitage

The Golden Rules of Travel

Plan your journey
Travel can be comfortable, fun, and relaxing, full of interest and excitement. To achieve this, you will need to plan your journey.

Prepare well
Enjoy planning your travel. Book well in advance, to avoid disappointment. Leave yourself plenty of time to get all the paperwork completed.

Travel light
Carry the minimum amount of luggage; use straps, backpacks and wheels to make life easier.

Insist on the detailed information you need
Draw up a list of questions before you telephone or call in at a travel agent or booking office. Make sure they are all answered fully.

Look after yourself
Your aim must be to travel in comfort, matching what you wear to the conditions. Travelling makes you hungry, so make sure you always have something on hand to eat and drink.

Be money wise
Take out insurance cover and don't offer easy pickings to thieves.

Choose the right way to go
Establish the best method of travelling in terms of cost, comfort and time.

Take your time
Enjoy your trip. If you have planned and prepared well there should be no need to hurry.

You can do it!
No trip is impossible (well, virtually none).

PART 2

Choosing the right way to go

In theory, getting from one place to another has never been easier. In practice, you need good quality information to make sure a journey is economical, comfortable and practical. In this part of the guide, we look at different ways of travelling, to help you choose the right way to go. We also look at things associated with travelling, such as getting to hospital or taking your pet on a journey. For easy reference, they are listed alphabetically.

AIR TRAVEL

Graham Lightfoot

Planning

Statistics show that air travel is a very safe way to get about the globe. Most airports have been designed around the needs of the business executive: they tend to be very modern, and organised so that checking-in and collecting baggage, getting passengers onto planes or out of the airport, is all done as swiftly as possible. Yet even those of us who have flown many times need to think carefully about all the different aspects of travelling by plane.

If you live near an airport and you have never travelled by air before, then a visit will enable you to become familiar with its layout (car parking, setting down point for taxis, location of luggage trolleys, domestic and international check-in desks) and the procedure for checking in. Even if your first flight is from another airport, you will at least have an idea of what to expect. Alternatively, ask your travel agent to describe the one you are going to (most good agents make a point of trying out the facilities they book their clients into).

Airports produce very comprehensive guides with layout plans and surface transport connections. For example, guides for many British airports (Aberdeen, Edinburgh, Gatwick, Glasgow, Heathrow, Prestwick and Stansted) are available from the British Airports Authority (see p 151).

Airlines and destinations

In order to find out which airlines operate to your destination a few options are open to you:

- check with your local travel agent
- phone your nearest airport (look under 'Airports and airfields' in Yellow Pages) to find out which airlines fly from it and, possibly, where they go

- phone the airline listed in Yellow Pages, under 'Airlines'
- ask any friends who have flown there before (if there is a choice of airline their opinions may be very relevant)

Economics

Although some airlines offer special fares for senior citizens, such fares are not necessarily the cheapest available. It pays to plan ahead as the cheapest fares are usually the ones with the most restrictions and need to be booked well in advance. These fares include Advance Purchase Excursion fares (known as APEX, SUPER APEX, PEX, SUPER PEX), and Advanced Booking Charter fares (known as ABC).

In order to secure cheap fares a number of conditions often apply:

- both the outward and the return portions of the journey have to be booked and paid for at the same time
- no alterations are permitted unless a higher fare is paid
- little or no refund for cancellation
- they are only available on certain days of the week or times of the year
- the minimum and maximum length of stay is fixed
- only a small number are available on each flight

It is essential when buying such tickets that you also take out insurance to cover you against the risk of having to cancel.

Clearly, your travel agent can steer you through the multitude of options, but friends who are experienced air travellers may also be a useful source of advice. In addition, discount tickets are also advertised in both local and national newspapers, which can be checked in the local library.

Many of these discount tickets are sold through so called 'bucket shops', which have bought them in bulk from the airlines themselves. Both the airlines and the 'bucket shops' are technically operating outside international aviation agreements, though it is perfectly legal for you to purchase such tickets from them. However, it is necessary to take certain precautions when buying tickets in this way, because the usual legal protection may not be available:

Check that you are getting a bargain by making some comparison with the cheap fares that are available elsewhere.

Make sure that you are happy with the airline concerned.

Check the restrictions applied to the ticket, so that you can change reservations if necessary.

Before you receive the ticket, pay only a small deposit, say 10 per cent and use a credit card for all payments, as this will give you protection under the Consumer Credit Act.

Phone the airline's reservation office to check your booking has been recorded correctly and confirm the return flight as soon as you reach your outward destination.

For large countries such as the USA, it is possible to purchase Air Passes, which give unlimited travel for a specified period on internal flights. Travel is however restricted to flights by the airline from which you bought the pass which means you often have to pass through one particular 'holiday' airport, on every flight you take. The best value pass usually has to be purchased in advance, in Britain. You will have to specify your flights (date, time and destination). However, once you have arrived in the United States, a phone call to the airline can usually get the whole schedule rearranged, so a pass is more flexible than it seems.

A recent development which can enable you to travel free on British Airways flights is the 'Air Miles' scheme. In order to participate in this scheme you have to become a registered Air Miles collector (Telephone: 0293 513633 for information). Air Miles can be collected by purchasing goods and services from the many shops and suppliers participating in the scheme and displaying the Air Miles logo. Every Air Mile collected is worth one mile of free travel with British Airways to international destinations served by the airline. The Air Miles brochure, which you are sent as a registered collector, lists the destinations served and the number of Air Miles required for a free scheduled ticket.

Choosing the right way to go

If you are flying abroad, even as far as Australia, you do not always have to fly from South East England (Heathrow, Gatwick, Luton or Stansted). Other airports (such as Birmingham International, Glasgow and Manchester) now have direct flights to a variety of destinations or can connect you with flights from there to your final destination airport. You can therefore avoid having to make lengthy surface journeys, which might include going across London.

Your travel agent, who has a directory of all flights from all airports, can often help you to decide the best one to fly from and to. For example, if you are flying to Australia or New Zealand you may prefer to travel via the USA rather than via the Middle East and Asia. In some cases it might be better to fly to somewhere outside the UK in order to get a better connection for intercontinental flights.

National Express (see p 153) operate direct coach services from many urban centres to most major airports, as does a Birmingham company called Flightlink (see p 151). There are bus and coach links between certain rail stations and most major airports. London Heathrow is served by the Underground. London Gatwick and Birmingham International are served by British Rail. Manchester Airport has a frequent Express Shuttle coach service from the two main railway stations. Belfast City Airport is served by Northern Ireland Railways. Most major airports in Britain are close to the motorway network.

If travel by public transport to and from the airport does not appeal to you and you are unwilling or unable to drive yourself there, try asking a friend or relative to take you there and meet you on your return. Remember to tell them your date and time of arrival and, most important of all, the flight number, so they can check whether it will be landing on time. Airports will quote times using the 24-hour clock and so a flight scheduled to arrive at three o'clock will land in the early hours of the morning.

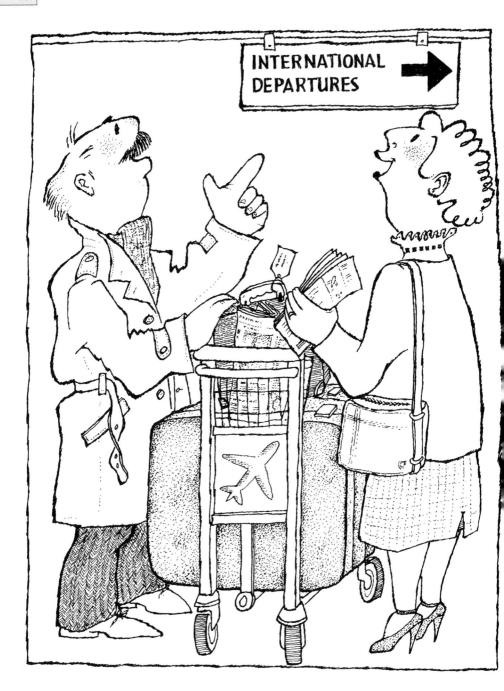

Making a booking

The most common way to book your flight is either through a travel agency or with the airline you have chosen. Besides the standard questions (see the Checklist in Part 1, Planning, on page 19), there are a number of things to remember to ask about:

Make sure that you have decided which airport (not just which city) you are leaving from and going to (many major cities have more than one).

Insist on seat allocation at the time of booking. For example in the no smoking areas or next to the emergency exit where there is usually more leg room.

Ask about latest (and earliest) check-in times.

Obtain clear information about airports and terminals.

Ask whether meals are served and order any special meals.

Luggage

The amount of luggage you can take depends upon the allowance shown on your ticket. This is usually determined by weight, but in some circumstances the number of pieces is limited. A good guide is one for the hold and one for the cabin. The latter must be able to fit under your seat and the total of the three dimensions (height, length and breadth) must not exceed 115cms (45 inches). In addition you can also carry the following items free of charge:

- handbag
- camera
- pair of binoculars
- overcoat
- cloak
- blanket
- umbrella
- walking stick
- some reading material

SOME USEFUL HINTS

- don't overpack your suitcase
- remove all labels from previous journeys
- strap your suitcase tightly and lock it
- put a distinguishing mark (use coloured tape) on the outside
- put only your destination address on the outside
- put your home address on a card inside (only put it outside on the return journey)
- make a list of the contents and keep it with you (you will need it should your baggage be lost and you make a claim)
- pack your toilet bag and a set of underwear in your cabin bag, just in case your suitcase is mislaid

Don't pack the following in your hold baggage: money, passport, tickets, credit cards, cheque book, traveller's cheques, jewellery, cameras, medicines, spectacles, keys, documents and any other valuable, fragile or irreplaceable items; in addition, any electronic equipment must have the batteries removed.

It is not advisable to carry on you or in your cabin baggage items such as scissors, knives or needles as they can be considered to be potential weapons and will probably be confiscated for the duration of the flight.

If your journey involves changing planes en route, then make sure that you can check your luggage through to your final destination airport, so that you don't need to worry about it during the change of planes.

There is a range of items which you must not take on an aircraft. These include:

- explosives: fireworks, flares, toy gun caps
- compressed gases: gas cylinders, aerosols other than medicinal or toilet articles
- flammable liquids and solids: lighter fuel, non-safety matches, paints, thinners, fire lighters
- oxidisers: some bleaching powders

- organic peroxides: some types of solid hydrogen peroxide
- poisons: arsenic, cyanide, weed-killer
- irritants: tear gas devices
- infectious substances: live viruses, bacteria
- radioactive materials: medical or research samples containing radioactive sources
- corrosives: acids, alkalis, wet cell type car batteries, caustic soda
- magnetised materials: magnetrons, instruments containing magnets
- miscellaneous: quicksilver, instruments containing mercury, quick lime, creosote, oiled paper.

If you are in any doubt about anything you wish to carry, then discuss it with the airline concerned.

Look after yourself

Ideally wear loose fitting clothing and comfortable soft shoes. Your feet can swell during a flight, so loosen your shoes, but don't take them off as you may find it difficult to get them back on.

On short flights there may be some light refreshments, and on longer flights there will be a full meal service, included in your ticket price. If you have ordered a special meal, make sure that the cabin crew are aware of this.

Travel by plane causes dehydration because of the air conditioning, so it is advisable to drink plenty during a flight. It is unwise to drink alcohol, as this will also contribute to your dehydration and it can have more effect than at ground level.

During take-off and landing your ears and nose will tend to feel blocked up. A way of combating this is to suck boiled sweets; some airlines hand them round just before take-off. It is always worth having your own supply; it is also one way of breaking the ice with other passengers.

Frailty and disability

If you have a disability or feel that you would like some assistance during your journey, then it is important that you make this clear at the time of booking. Specify the nature of your disability and the assistance required at all stages of the journey. You need to check that all the facilities you require are definitely available and that you can travel unaccompanied if you intend to travel alone.

If you are a wheelchair user, then check that you can go in your wheelchair right up to the aircraft; this is usually only possible if you have a manual chair and this can be stowed in the hold for immediate use at the destination. You can take your wheelchair at no extra charge and provided certain conditions are met powered wheelchairs can also be taken. In order to avoid the loss of or damage to removable parts of your wheelchair take them as hand luggage.

If you use crutches or any other device to assist you, then these travel at no extra charge. For those with a visual impairment, it is important to note that at many airports boarding announcements are now only made on the television monitors.

For those with hearing impairments, some of the major airports have now installed induction loop systems. In addition, some of the airline and airport staff may be proficient in signing.

At all major airports it is possible to make use of small powered carts to avoid the long walks which are a common feature. These have to be ordered in advance.

Most airlines will insist upon some form of medical clearance before accepting people with disabilities as passengers. In order to simplify this process, a standard form (MEDIF) has been produced for completion by the booking agent and your doctor; and for frequent travellers a card (FREMEC) is available free of charge. British Airways (see p 151) publish a guide for doctors entitled *Your Patient and Air Travel* and also a set of leaflets (see Further Reading p 52).

The major airports are now designed or adapted to cater for people who require assistance, and facilities such as lifts, mobile walkways and wheelchair-accessible toilets are common features. The guides issued by the airport management contain details of all these facilities.

Some of the larger so-called 'wide-bodied aircraft' have wheelchairs on board and other aircraft are equipped with carrying chairs.

If you have a mobility handicap, try to ensure that you are seated near to the toilets on the aircraft. Check with your travel agent what arrangements need to be made before travelling.

Common problems

If you miss your flight or connection, even though you may have the most restricted ticket available, it is quite likely that you will be allowed to 'standby' for the next available flight to your chosen destination.

Sometimes flights are overbooked, because the airlines always try to fill their planes and there will always be some people who book on more than one flight. Very rarely, even though your ticket is valid, you can be denied carriage. Fortunately, there is a set procedure that most scheduled airlines adhere to, which entails putting you on another flight due to arrive at your destination within a set time of your original flight or paying you compensation if this is not possible.

If your luggage is mislaid, it will either turn up on the next flight or soon after. If you have followed the tips outlined you will manage in the meantime without it. In the event of outright loss, you will have to claim on your insurance.

If you have checked in for your flight and gone through passport control you can still take out insurance cover. At most airports there is a kiosk 'airside' where you can obtain insurance cover, although it may be a bit more expensive than your local broker.

At both London Heathrow and London Gatwick there is an independent social work agency, Travel Care (see p 151), which can offer support if you have a problem or need help in an emergency.

FURTHER READING

- *Care in the Air,* available free from Air Transport Users Committee – advice for handicapped travellers.

- *Flight plan,* available free from Air Transport Users Committee – hints for airline passengers.

- *Personal Toilet on Long Flights,* published by Disabled Living Foundation, single copies for personal use are free.

- *The Complete Sky Traveller,* by David Beaty, published by Methuen, price £2.95.

- *The Round the World Air Guide,* by Katie Wood and George McDonald, published by Fontana, price £10.99.

- *Travel Wise,* a set of leaflets from British Airways, including the following:

  First Time Traveller

  Travelling as an Elderly Passenger

  Incapacitated Passengers

  Dangerous Articles in Baggage

  Cabin Baggage

  Special Meals

BUSES
Caroline Cahm and Michael Dearing

Bus travel still represents good value for money even though, like all goods and services, bus fares have risen quite significantly in recent years. On journeys of up to about 15 miles you will pay less than travelling by train, yet as long as you travel outside peak hours the journey times will not be that much different.

Concessionary travel

The level of concession made available to bus users (bus passes or tokens), is generally at the discretion of the local authority. Borough, district and in some cases county councils or Passenger Transport Executives administer these essentially local schemes and it is they who decide on the type and value of the concessionary travel provided in their area, and make arrangements for any necessary passes or tokens to be issued.

Many of them have separate schemes for older people and for people with a disability of some kind, which may include epilepsy, partial sight, and so on. If you qualify under both schemes, get their details to compare which one will benefit you most. It is very important that you find out from your local authority what limitations there are with your local travel schemes. Some bus companies in your area may not be included and there may be restrictions when you travel into the area of another local authority.

Although there is no national scheme for pensioners, men over 65 and women over 60 qualify for some form of concessionary travel in almost all areas of the country. Broadly speaking, there are four types of scheme:

1 Travel tokens of a set value, issued each year. These can be used for part or full payment of fares and in some cases can be used to purchase Senior Railcards, and so on.

2 A pass giving flat rate for any length of journey on one bus in a

given area.

3 A half fare bus pass, usually limited to off-peak travel Mondays to Fridays, but which can be used at any time at weekends and on public holidays.

4 A pass giving completely free bus travel but again often limited to off-peak, weekend and public holiday journeys.

There is considerable variation in what is provided from one district to another. You may be able to use a half-fare pass to travel to a town in a neighbouring authority's area as long as you do not have to change buses on the way – but not if you want to make a further journey in your destination area. Again, as there is no national scheme for cheap bus travel, your pass will almost certainly not be valid if you travel to a distant town for a holiday or to visit relatives.

In addition, a number of bus operators have their own cheap travel schemes for pensioners including half fare passes, discounted travel cards and multi-journey tickets.

Comfort and convenience

But even if bus travel is relatively cheap with concessionary fares, is it always an easy and comfortable way to get about? Undoubtedly there have been problems here. Outside London, the bus operators long ago converted their fleets to one-person operation – a change which led to the loss of the conductor, who was available to assist the less nimble to board and alight.

The only substantial investment in new buses (until comparatively recently) has been associated with the widespread introduction of minibuses on urban networks. Unfortunately these vehicles have provided less satisfactory access and less space for shopping trolleys and luggage than the big buses they replaced. However, they do have the advantage that they often go right into housing estates, and many operate on a hail-and-ride basis – letting you catch them much nearer home.

The good news is that the latest single and double decker buses coming into service are designed with features that make getting on and off the bus and moving about inside easier for everyone. Also, a number of operators are adapting existing buses to make them more 'user friendly', for instance, by adding brightly coloured and easy to hold grab rails. The first generation minibuses (which were only conversions of standard delivery vans) are now being replaced by purpose-built midibuses, equipped with:

- wider doorways
- lower floors and/or less steep steps
- wider gangways
- more space for shopping
- less cramped seating

In addition, there is a growing number of routes covered by buses equipped with a passenger lift or a ramp, and the facility to carry passengers in wheelchairs. These are often marketed under special names such as Mobility Buses, Care Buses, Access Buses, Local Line and Easy Rider.

The routes generally give a passenger the opportunity to travel once or twice a week into town to do shopping or carry out other business, and often go past hospitals, clinics and sheltered accommodation. All such services are subsidised, so your local transport authority will be able to give you the relevant details.

Finally, in some parts of the country, the conductor is being reintroduced, or else special voluntary 'bus helpers' are recruited, whose duty it is to help people onto and off the bus, to and from their seat, deal with shopping and luggage, and so on.

Bus information

You may well have to make an effort to get accurate up-to-date information about the times, routes and destinations of your local bus services.

The main operators in your area will publish timetable booklets or leaflets for all the commercial services, contracted services and journeys they run themselves, even though they may not include details of journeys being provided by other companies.

Local authorities often distribute timetable leaflets and books to local public libraries and tourist information offices. Some county councils, regional councils (in Scotland) and Passenger Transport Executives (in metropolitan areas) also publish comprehensive timetable booklets for particular localities or even timetable books covering all bus services in their area. Much of the timetable information is free but in some cases there will be a charge, particularly where a general guide for the whole area is provided. Nearly all bus operators have provision for enquiries about bus times and fares by telephone.

In addition, a visit to a bus enquiry or booking office will also give you the opportunity of picking up not only timetable booklets or leaflets but also leaflets giving details of special fares promotions, day tours and coach holidays. Some, but not all, publish useful route maps – very helpful for a newcomer and giving ideas for trips by bus for both residents and holiday-makers.

'Explorer' tickets

Armed with a route map and details of special fares offers, it is possible to plan days out by service bus. A popular ticket to buy in the provinces is the 'Explorer' ticket; most of the major bus companies sell this type of ticket which gives unlimited travel for a day, and usually not only on their buses but on those of neighbouring operators too. In the South East, for example, the 'Explorer' day ticket currently costs £3.50 (£2.50 for pensioners) and is valid on the buses of all major operators in Kent, Hampshire, and East and West Sussex . 'Explorer' tickets can be purchased in advance at bus travel offices or from the driver on the first bus you board on the day of your trip. The bus travel office staff will give you any help you require in planning your day out and you will often find that it is possible to travel to your selected destination by one route and return by another and, of course, you can break your journey either out or back to spend an hour or so at another place of interest.

Catching the bus

Always signal clearly that you want the bus to stop, particularly if you live in an area where the bus company operates a 'hail and ride' system, where there are no fixed bus stops. You can help the bus driver by having your pass and money ready when you board. Do not be afraid to ask the driver to give you time to get to a seat before the bus sets off and, if you are going to an unfamiliar destination, ask for a call when the bus arrives there.

To make a success of any bus journey, it is important to plan in advance and this goes just as much for a trip to the local shops as it does for a whole day out with an 'Explorer' ticket. Check the bus times both ways and be at the stop with a few minutes to spare. Be sure to avoid long waits at bus stops, especially if the weather is not very good.

Avoid travelling at the busier times if at all possible, that is, when work people or school children are likely to be travelling. Not only will the bus be less crowded but the driver will have more time to give you any information or assistance that you require. Do not be afraid to try longer bus journeys, especially where the route takes you through pleasant rural areas; you see much more of the countryside from a bus than from a private car and the slower speed ensures that you miss nothing.

Take things calmly, plan your journey in advance and enjoy it.

CARS See section on Money page 35

Michelle Le Prevost

For many drivers, running a car can offer them the road to independence, particularly if their personal mobility is limited in some way. Cars can certainly make door-to-door trips easier, but if you only need this type of transport for a hospital appointment or weekly shopping, a taxi could prove more economical (see Example 3 in Part 1, Money, on page 36).

You do not need to own a car to have use of one. Many formal and informal car-sharing schemes operate across the country, where a friend or neighbour can provide car transport for a contribution towards the petrol costs. Some community groups run car services for essential journeys (see Community Transport section on page 82). Ask about local services at your Citizens Advice Bureau.

Car hire

Cars can be hired from a range of national, regional and local companies, all of whom should be listed in your local Yellow Pages. If a choice exists, the firm chosen should be a member of the British Vehicle Rental and Leasing Association (BVRLA) (see p 151).

Before hiring a car, check out any 'extras' not included in the basic hire charge; typically, motor insurance and personal accident insurance will be additional, as will VAT. Some companies make additional charges for mileage or require you to return the vehicle with a full tank of fuel. Many companies now insist on a (returnable) deposit. If you have time, get quotations from a number of firms before making your choice.

You may not be able to use your own motor insurance cover when driving a hired vehicle, so be sure to check any restrictions imposed by the car hirers' insurers, especially if you want to hire a large-engined vehicle or share the driving with another passenger. Take care, as some car hire insurance companies surcharge or severely restrict older drivers.

When you arrive to pick up the car, do not forget to have your driving licence available for inspection (they will want to see this every time you hire a car). If the car you booked is unavailable (the previous driver might have extended their hire), you may be offered a more expensive car instead: insist on paying at the rate of the one you booked.

How much will running a car cost me?

If you have a car already, then it can be very helpful to keep a small book in the car to record journeys made, and expenditure. For the cost of a few seconds writing down the information, you will get a good idea of your miles per gallon, by looking at the mileage undertaken and comparing it with the cost of fuel used. If this is below average for your car, or if it drops from a previous figure, it probably means that your car needs a service. The information will also help you forecast what you will have to spend in the future.

An annual budget for your car is quite easy to work out (see also Example 3 on page 36) and comprises the following elements:

■ Road Fund Licence (Vehicle Excise Duty)

■ insurance (take into account any no claims bonus and special deals you may get for being an older driver; make sure you insure the car comprehensively)

■ cleaning (car wash, or the cost of wax and shampoo if you do it yourself)

■ fuel (if you keep records of your journeys and expenditure, then working this out will be easy; otherwise, estimate how many miles you will do in a year, and divide this by an average miles per gallon figure for your car, to get the number of gallons of fuel you will use; multiply this by the average cost of a gallon of fuel, to get the total cost of fuel in the year)

■ servicing and maintenance (the older the car gets, the more it will cost to service; new cars may have free service for the first one or two years, but not all parts may be covered by such deals, and generally you will still have to pay for oil and so on; it is unlikely that this figure will cost much less than 3p per mile)

- motoring organisation membership
- miscellaneous (eg de-icer, parking costs, accessories)
- depreciation (strictly speaking, this is not a cost, as you do not have to pay anything out to anyone; however, it is here to remind you that most cars go down in value as you use them; to make up the difference between what you would get for your old car, and the cost of a new car, you will either have to raid your capital, or else have put some money by on a regular basis)

People on lower incomes have difficulty meeting large and unexpected bills. If you do a budget as outlined above, then it tells you how much you will need to save each month for the large annual payments such as insurance and road fund licence. In addition, it may be possible to spread the payments out more. Insurance can generally be paid for in instalments, and you can buy six months road fund licence at a time.

You can spend less on your car, in a wide variety of ways:

If it is a petrol engined car, then make sure it is converted to use unleaded petrol. In addition to reducing the pollution in the air, it will reduce your fuel bill by at least 5 per cent.

Make sure the engine is properly serviced. Poorly adjusted engines will use up much more fuel than necessary.

Try not using the car for short journeys – if it is possible walk instead.

Do some of your own maintenance. Not everyone wants to wield a spanner, but most of us can manage to check and top up the oil, water, and other fluids, and put batteries on charge. Just doing this will save you money. To learn more about this, an evening class in basic car maintenance will be very helpful.

Drive smoothly, with a light right foot. Harsh braking, cornering and acceleration costs money. Take your time.

If the time comes to replace your car, get a smaller one. This is particularly true if you are losing the company car on retirement.

Unless you really need electric windows and central locking, get the basic model – it is much cheaper. Diesel engined cars are cheaper to run, need less maintenance and use less (and cheaper) fuel. However, they cost more to buy, so you have to calculate whether you will save this extra amount within the lifetime of the car. Those doing low mileage should probably stick to petrol engined cars.

Share the costs. If you are going out with friends, don't take two separate cars. Take it in turns to give each other lifts.

The overall cost will depend to a great extent on the number of miles you drive each year and the size of the engine in your car. In the case of a new car with an engine capacity up to 2000 cc, the Automobile Association (see p 150) reckon the following costs (depreciation included) apply:

MILEAGE	PENCE PER MILE		
	Unleaded petrol	Leaded petrol	Diesel
5,000 miles	59.230	59.663	49.823
10,000 miles	36.832	37.265	30.838
15,000 miles	31.287	31.720	26.041
20,000 miles	29.956	30.389	22.494
25,000 miles	29.157	29.590	22.203
30,000 miles	26.703	27.136	20.478

Ref   The Automobile Association, April 1990
Note   Significant changes in the price of fuel will inevitably affect these figures.

What to look for when buying a car

Your first choice may well be between a new car or a second-hand one. New cars are more expensive but carry a warranty from the manufacturer and repair and maintenance costs should be lower, at least for the first three years. If you are considering buying a used car, look for a low mileage vehicle with a record of regular servicing (ask to see the receipts for parts). It is always wise to get the vehicle checked by someone with technical knowledge. Most of the motoring organisations provide this type of service.

Most drivers want the same from their car: reliability, comfort, performance and economy. However, it is important to consider not just your needs now, but how those needs may change in the next few years. If you carry a passenger regularly, their needs must be taken into consideration also.

Many models are available with automatic transmission, power steering or servo-assisted brakes, all of which can make life easier for the driver. Electric controls reduce the amount of physical effort required and central locking has obvious advantages.

Whether you choose a saloon or estate car will depend largely on your need to carry luggage or bulky items, on a regular basis. Consider whether a large car might be more difficult to park. A reasonable compromise could be a hatchback, but be careful: check the height of the sill and the reach required to get things in and out over the bumper.

It is most important for anyone who uses a wheelchair or walking aid to take it with them when they test drive a car. Check that it can be stowed easily and securely.

As far as the actual dimensions of the car are concerned, you must be able to get in and out of the car easily. Some aspects to look for are:

Door width
A two door car usually has wider doors because there is no need for a central doorpost. You should check the grip on the door handles and the amount of reach required to close the door once it is fully extended.

Low door sill
The lower the sill, the less the knees have to be lifted to step into the car.

Shallow floor well
The distance between the door sill and the car floor, dictates the amount of bending required to get out of the vehicle.

Seat height
Low seats require more effort and more bending, higher seats reduce

this, but may increase the chance of hitting your head on the door frame.

Door frame height

This will be relative to the driver's height. Too low a frame will mean you will have to stoop to get into the car.

Central console

Some drivers prefer to enter the car from the passenger side and slide across. In this case the design of the central console will be very important.

Some fairly minor modifications can be made, to make life easier:

Seat runners can be extended, to allow the seat to be pushed right back for easier entrance or exit.

Inertia reel seat belts are unsatisfactory for anyone with weak arms, so an alternative could be a static belt or harness.

Seat belt extensions are a simple answer to 'difficult-to-reach' belts; similarly a tension device can be useful to anyone who feels 'choked' by their seatbelt. Both of these devices are generally available from good motor accessories shops. Under certain circumstances exemption from wearing your seatbelt can be obtained. For more information, speak to your family doctor.

Additional handles or detachable gripping devices can be useful for someone with weak legs, but who still has strength in their arms. Your local garage can fit extra handles above the door or to the door pillar for you. Similarly your local garage may be able to fit a doorstop, which prevents the car door from swinging shut whilst you are trying to get in or out.

Modifications to the existing seat runners so that the seats can swivel through 90 degrees, enabling you to sit on them outside the car.

Breakdown

If you are planning a long trip in the car, it would be worth considering what you would do if your vehicle broke down. A little thought before you leave home could prevent problems later. Check the general condition of your car, including tyre pressure and tread, oil, fuel, and water levels. Top up if necessary.

Invest in membership of a reliable breakdown and recovery service. If you are a wheelchair user or have other special needs, check that the breakdown service you have chosen can fully cater for your needs. A full list of breakdown/recovery services can be found in the Yellow Pages. Most cars come equipped with enough tools to change a tyre. You might like to buy a warning triangle and a tow rope to complete the kit.

If your vehicle does break down, the chances are you will lose both light and heat. A good torch in the glove compartment and a blanket on the back seat are essential items. A thermos of tea or soup is always a good standby even if you intend to stop and eat en route. If you have a medical condition that means you must eat or drink regularly, be particularly sure to pack something in case of emergency.

Frailty and disability

For some people an illness or the onset of some disability may force them to give up driving, at least for a while. If you are returning to driving after a while or are unsure of your ability to continue driving, there are now a number of centres where you can undertake a driving assessment. Most centres make some charge but nearly all offer a range of adapted vehicles to demonstrate that disability or infirmity need not be a barrier to getting back on the road. A full list of assessment centres can be obtained from the Department of Transport's Mobility Advice and Vehicle Information Service (MAVIS) (see p 152).

A lot of older or disabled travellers will need to stop for the toilet at regular intervals. Plan your journey with this in mind. Specialised toileting aids are available for those with a special need. Your doctor or district nurse will be able to advise you.

Motability

Motability is a non-profit making voluntary organisation that was formed when the Mobility Allowance was introduced. The aim of the organisation is to help people wishing to buy a car or wheelchair to spend their Mobility Allowance to their best advantage. Motability is able to negotiate discounts with car and wheelchair manufacturers as well as insurance companies and motoring organisations. In the past ten years Motability has provided more than 100,000 cars for disabled people.

There are two ways that you can obtain a new car through Motability:

1 The Motability Hire Scheme

Anyone in receipt of a Mobility Allowance, that has more than three years to run, can obtain a car this way. You do not have to be the driver to apply. Also parents can obtain a car this way for a child who is receiving Mobility Allowance.

Hirers select from a list of 250 models, with maintenance, servicing and AA membership inclusive in the charge. In addition, hire car users get free 'loss of use' cover, giving them a weekly sum, if the vehicle is off the road for any reason.

Hirers pay an advance payment and then a fixed weekly rental. In addition, you have to pay for any adaptations and the cost of removing them at the end of the three year hiring period.

Under the hire scheme, a mileage charge is levied on anyone who exceeds 12,000 miles a year. However, if the total mileage over the three year period is less than 36,000 miles, the mileage charge will be refunded.

Other costs include a contribution towards your insurance premium and of course, the vehicle running costs.

Motability has a charitable fund for anyone who is unable to afford the advance payments or the extra cost of adaptations, but there is a waiting list.

2 The Hire Purchase Scheme

The eligibility rules for buying your own car under the Hire Purchase Scheme are the same as for the Hire Scheme, except your

Mobility Allowance must have at least four years to run. Virtually any new model can be bought this way, but if you choose a model that isn't listed, you may have to negotiate the price with the dealer yourself.

Under the Hire Purchase Scheme you need to pay for Fully Comprehensive insurance cover (which you need to arrange yourself), running costs, maintenance and servicing, and motoring organisation membership. In addition, you pay a deposit on the vehicle and regular HP instalments. The Hire Purchase can be arranged over a four, four and a half, or five year period.

Motability can undertake purchase of a second-hand vehicle that has passed an inspection, providing the buyer's Mobility Allowance has at least two years to run.

A.I.D. *Assistance and Independence for the Disabled*

A.I.D. offer a selection of quality used cars to disabled people. You do not have to be in receipt of Mobility Allowance to be eligible. A.I.D. prepare all the vehicles in their own workshops and are able to offer warranty cover. Adaptations and accessories can also be fitted before delivery. Home delivery of the vehicle to anywhere on the U.K. mainland is provided free of charge.

Choice of vehicle is from their current stocks, but A.I.D. will try to locate a suitable vehicle to meet the needs of the individual driver. Purchase of the vehicle can be in cash, through your own finance arrangement, or through A.I.D.'s own finance plan.

Insurance

The cost of your insurance will depend on a number of factors: the type of cover, the type of car, the area where you live, your age and your previous driving record.

Insurance companies who feel they have not been given the full facts may invalidate claims made against them. Drivers have a responsibility to declare to their insurance company any disability they may have or any adaptations made to their vehicle.

Some insurance companies will charge more for disabled or older drivers, whilst others charge less, so shop around for quotes before you decide on a policy. An insurance broker may well be able to provide you with a choice of policies.

Make sure you have adequate cover. Third party cover is the legal minimum but will not cover injury to you or damage to your car. Comprehensive policies are the best, and strongly recommended for owners of new cars, but invariably cost more. Whatever type of cover you choose, read the policy document in detail before you sign.

A list of brokers and agents who specialise in policies for older and disabled drivers appears at the end of this section.

Driving licences

Many drivers worry about their ability to drive as they get older. The law states that anyone with a 'relevant' or 'prospective' disability may have their licence refused, revoked or limited. 'Relevant' disabilities include:

- epilepsy
- severe mental handicap
- giddiness or fainting attacks
- inability to read a registration plate at a distance of 20.5 metres
- any other disability likely to cause danger to the public

'Prospective' disabilities tend to be either intermittent (happening from time-to-time) or progressive (gradually happening over a period of time) and may eventually become a 'relevant' disability.

Anyone applying for a licence is legally bound to declare any disability, whether relevant or prospective. Similarly the onset of any disability, once a licence has been issued, must be notified to the DVLC in Swansea (see p 152). Temporary disabilities like a broken leg, are excluded from the ruling.

If you are in any doubt about your medical condition and think that it may affect your driving ability you should consult your doctor.

Additional information about relevant and prospective disabilities can be found in leaflet D100, which is available at your Post Office.

When a licence is issued it will, depending on the fitness of the driver, be issued until the age of 70. After this, it will have to be renewed every three years. Normally the DVLC will send a reminder and renewal form (D46) eight weeks before the licence expires. If this does not arrive you can renew your licence using form D1 available from the Post Office. Any recent disability or medical condition must be declared on this form. The new licence may be reissued for a period of one, two or three years.

Vehicle Excise Duty *Road Tax*

Motor vehicles are subject to annual Road Tax. Under certain circumstances disabled drivers may be eligible for exemption. Application forms for Vehicle Excise Duty Exemption (MY181) are sent out by the DSS. If you receive Mobility Allowance or War Pensioners Mobility Supplement, you should get one automatically. The form should be completed and returned to the Mobility Allowance Unit at Blackpool (see DSS p 152).

The Mobility Unit will issue a certificate (MY182) which may be used to claim exemption from Road Tax. Exemption is not automatic and is at the discretion of the Department of Transport.

If you are applying for a vehicle licence for the first time you should use form V10 from your local Post Office. You will need all of the documents specified; vehicle registration document, insurance certificate and M.O.T. (if applicable). Post them with your MY182 certificate to your local Vehicle Registration Office. Their address is listed in the phone book under 'Transport, Department of'.

An exempt licence and exempt licence disc will be issued. The licence disc must be displayed in the car windscreen and renewed when it expires, in the same way as an ordinary tax disc. If you are renewing your licence, you will be sent a form from the DVLC. Renewal of exempt licences can be done at the Post Office.

If you are disabled but not in receipt of Mobility Allowance you may still be eligible for exemption. Further enquiries should be made to the DSS Disablement Services Branch (see p 152).

VAT exemption

If you are purchasing a vehicle specially designed or adapted for a disabled person, you may be eligible for zero-rating for VAT (Value Added Tax) on the purchase. So, you do not need to pay the VAT. This zero-rating also applies to repairs and spare parts for the vehicle.

When you are making your purchase, you should make it clear that your purchase will be zero rated for VAT. This is very important as you cannot reclaim the VAT once it has been paid. If necessary, you may be asked to sign a form declaring your exemption.

More information is available from the local VAT Office, listed in the phone book under H.M. Customs and Excise.

The Orange Badge Scheme

The Orange Badge Scheme is a national arrangement to allow on-street parking for disabled and blind people. It is currently under review, so you should check whether new arrangements have been introduced.

You do not need to own a car, or be the driver, to apply for an Orange Badge, as it may be displayed in the windscreen of any car in which the holder travels.

You are eligible for an Orange Badge if:

- you receive Mobility Allowance
- you are blind
- you use a Government supplied vehicle
- you are unable to walk or have severe difficulty in walking (in this case you will need to supply medical confirmation of your condition)

If you think you may be eligible for an Orange Badge you should apply to your local social services department. If you live in Scotland, you should apply to the Chief Executive of your regional council.

There are certain areas where the Orange Badge Scheme does not apply, these are:

- some airports, eg Heathrow
- some town centres
- areas limited to vehicles with special permits
- central London boroughs where parking problems are acute (here the Green Badge Scheme operates)

The Orange Badge entitles the holder to:

- park without charge or limit at parking meters
- park without time limit where only limited waiting is normally allowed
- park for up to two hours on single or double yellow lines in England and Wales, and without time limit in Scotland
- park wherever local authorities have made special arrangements for Orange Badge holders

The Green Badge Scheme

Orange Badges may not be used in the central London boroughs of the City of London, the City of Westminster, the Royal Borough of Kensington and Chelsea, and some parts of the Borough of Camden. In these areas a separate Green Badge Scheme operates for disabled local residents and employees.

The Green Badge entitles the holder to park without charge or limit at parking meters, resident parking spaces and designated disabled areas. It does not allow parking on yellow lines.

Applications for Green Badges should be made to the London borough where you need to park as each of the boroughs operates its own scheme.

Motoring holidays

Motoring holidays offer a great deal in terms of independence and flexibility, but the secret to a good motoring holiday is in the planning.

Start planning your holiday well in advance, so you are not rushing around at the last minute, or leaving things to chance. Make sure that you have suitable insurance, not just to cover the vehicle, but in case of accident to yourself or your passenger.

Any kind of 'get-you-home' motor cover is essential. All the good motoring organisations offer this type of service. If you are travelling abroad, your insurance company will usually supply a 'green card' to extend the cover of your motor insurance. Remember to contact them in plenty of time or they will charge you extra for arranging cover in a hurry. More specialist protection can be obtained to give you on-the-spot assistance in a foreign country.

Roll-on roll-off ferries now operate from a large number of ports offering a gateway to Europe. Many offer discounts to disabled drivers. Other travellers should look out for economy fares. Many camping firms, which supply pre-erected tents complete with beds and fully-equipped kitchens, have their own arrangements with the ferry companies, and offer good value packages.

Motorail

What could be a more simple start to your holiday than having your car loaded onto a Motorail train and then enjoying your (overnight) journey in comfort? Whether you choose a sleeper or a seat, additional assistance is available to get you there from your car, if you require it. You should contact the area manager at your departure station in good time.

The Motorail network operates across the country with services from London Euston (to Aberdeen, Carlisle, Edinburgh, and Inverness), London Paddington (to Penzance), and Bristol (to Edinburgh).

Motorail can be an expensive option as there are few discounts available. An off-peak return for a car and driver from Paddington to Penzance is £175, with any accompanying passengers paying £59 (return). Railcard holders get a £10 discount. There are other discounts for holders of Disabled Persons' Railcards. However this type of journey could save you becoming very tired during a long journey, and the wear and tear on the car. Motorail offers links to similar systems in Europe.

Full details of Motorail services are available in a brochure available from British Rail Travel Centres and their agents, or from your motoring organisation.

Motorways

Planning a motorway journey needs extra care. Check your vehicle is in good condition and that you have catered for potential emergencies. Information about road conditions can be obtained in advance through the television Ceefax or Oracle services, or by British Telecom's 'Traveline' service. A summary of conditions on all the motorways and major trunk roads is available by dialling 071-246 8031. AA and RAC members can get up to the minute information on their route through the Roadwatch and Motoring Hotline services.

Service stations

All motorways have service station facilities. They are places to take some time to stop for a rest and freshen up or have a hot drink. Full facilities exist to give the car a quick service, remembering to check all fluid levels and to refuel.

All service stations now provide toilet facilities for disabled people and hot food available on the ground floor. However, if you want something more than a burger and a cup of tea in a polystyrene beaker, you could be faced with a number of steps up to the main restaurant. Not all service stations have customer lifts but most have goods lifts that they will allow customers to use.

If you have special needs or require assistance when you reach the motorway service station, you should contact them in advance to make arrangements. Telephone numbers for the motorway service stations can be obtained through Directory Enquiries by reference to the motorway number (eg M1).

FURTHER READING

■ *Ins and outs of car choice: A guide for elderly and disabled people,* published by the Department of Transport and available through HMSO, price £1.80 inc. p & p.

■ *Motoring and mobility for disabled people* by Ann Darnborough and Derek Kinrade, published by RADAR, price £5.00 inc p & p.

■ *The Highway Code,* published by the Department of Transport, available from HMSO and bookshops, price 60p.

■ *Which? Magazine,* has a regular separate section on cars and motoring costs, published by the Consumer Association.

COACHES

Ian Yearsley

'Ride the highway, see the by-way' was once the slogan of a local coach company, and it illustrates some of the advantages of coach travel. You are, in effect, chauffeur-driven, and you do not need to worry about driving or maintaining a vehicle. The seating is set higher than in a motor car, enabling you to see over hedges and get a good view of the road ahead.

Economics

Fares are cheaper than rail, generally speaking, and there is someone to turn to if you have problems: the driver, and sometimes a steward too. You do not have to walk the length of a train to find the guard. Your heavy luggage is safely stowed away for you, though this means you cannot get to it during the journey.

If you are travelling in a group, a coach can take you all together without worrying about who needs to travel in whose car, or the need for checks on second glasses of wine with dinner for the drivers. Coach travel also has a good safety record.

All new coaches are now fitted with speed limiters that govern the maximum speed of the coach to 70 mph, and other coaches built after April 1974 will have to have limiters by 1991.

As with many things, you get what you pay for. Fares are cheaper, but journey times are almost always longer than rail, and there is less space for each person in a coach than in most InterCity trains. But standards have improved considerably in recent years, and many long-distance coaches now have a washroom and toilet; some also have a pantry enabling a steward to serve drinks and snacks.

Well-developed network

Britain has one of the most well-developed networks of timetabled express coach services in Europe. Since 1980, coach operators have been allowed to compete, but most services are run by one or other of the large companies.

By far the largest is National Express (see p 153), with about 600 coaches in its distinctive white livery, it carries some 14 million passengers a year to 1,500 destinations in England, Wales and Scotland. The Scottish end of its network is known as Caledonian Express (see p 153), and was formerly the coaching network of the Perth-based company Stagecoach which continues to run local buses.

Most National Express vehicles, belong to local coach companies who supply them under contract, but all have to conform to its standards. In summer it hires in other coaches of the same quality, so that on busy days there may be as many as 900 coaches on the road.

The second largest network is that of Scottish Citylink (see p 153), which grew out of the coaching enterprise of companies in the Scottish Bus Group. Citylink acted as National Express's partner until the end of the 1980s; they now compete and have separate booking offices at London's Victoria Coach Station.

There are many independent coach operators with networks of a few routes, or even just one service. West Midlands Travel (see p 153), for instance, operates its Central-Liner Londonlink service from Birmingham, and Armstrong Galley (see p 153) runs from Newcastle-upon-Tyne to London (tickets sold in branches of W H Smith in London).

Making a booking

If you want to make a journey by coach you will need to find a travel agent who handles coach bookings (not all do) and ask about timings and fares. There are lists of travel agents in the Yellow Pages.

The agent will want to know what day of the week you want to travel. In summer, National Express offers economy return fares if you avoid travelling on Fridays both ways, and also avoid Saturdays in

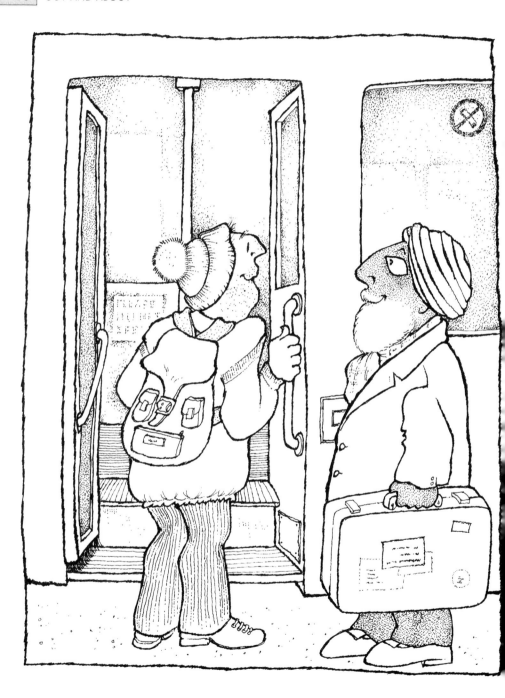

July and August. In winter (from October to April) there are also 'Boomerang' fares. They are 10 per cent cheaper still, if outward and return journeys are made on Tuesdays, Wednesdays or Saturdays.

Your agent will also ask whether you want a 'standard booking' or an 'assured reservation'. An assured reservation costs £1.20 regardless of the number of people on the ticket, but it assures everyone a seat on a particular departure. It must be made before the date of travel, and is advisable at busy times, for overnight journeys, and whenever it is important that the journey is made at a specific time, such as to a medical appointment. A standard booking provides travel on the date shown on the ticket, but does not guarantee a specific departure.

Accompanied children under five travel free, from five to fifteen at a concession rate, and there are discount cards for students. All men and women aged 60 or over are charged approximately two-thirds of the appropriate fare. Sometimes the agent or booking clerk will ask for evidence of age, such as a pension book, passport or driving licence, especially with people who look particularly youthful.

Tickets can be bought by credit card from most National Express telephone enquiry centres, but you need to allow at least five days for tickets to be processed and sent to you. There are some services, such as the Oxford-London and Green Line services, where there is no advance booking and you simply pay the driver, as on a bus. Some services run only once or twice a day, others every hour or half hour. But take care in booking, for some journeys may be direct, while others call at many places on the way. Scottish Citylink's London-Edinburgh service, for instance, has some direct routes, via the motorways, taking seven hours and fifty minutes, but there is a night-time service with 23 intermediate stops, taking eleven hours thirty minutes in all. Overnight coach journeys are more for the student, the young and the rugged person who can sleep on a seat as easily as in a bed. Again, if you do use them, look carefully at timings; do you really want to arrive somewhere at 6.30 am and then have to wait or walk around for an hour before you can find anywhere that will serve you breakfast?

To get the best out of the coach networks, travel at the quietest times of the week, usually Tuesdays and Wednesdays, when the lowest fares apply, and take advantage of the cheaper fares for the over-60s.

At the coach station

Most express coach services start and finish their journey at a coach station. Arriving in good time, and finding out where the coach will stand is, of course, part of your planning and preparation. It is also a chance to talk to other passengers going on the same departure.

Have your ticket ready to hand to the driver and he (or she) will take your heavy luggage (not more than one suitcase, preferably) and put it in the locker at the rear or nearside of the coach. Space is limited inside the coach, so take with you only what you absolutely need for the journey. The driver will return your luggage at your destination; if you are getting off before the final stop, tell the driver so that your luggage can be stowed near the front of the compartment.

Taking care of yourself

Most coach services stop every few hours at a motorway service area where there are toilets and refreshments. The driver will announce how long you are staying there; do not overstay this time or you will delay other passengers and you may even get left behind.

During the 1980s, National Express developed a new kind of up-market coach service on several routes, using coaches with toilets and with stewards serving light refreshments. Some of these are double deck coaches, and all are known as Rapides. Scottish Citylink designates such coaches as 'Cordon Bleu'; both networks charge a slightly higher fare for these services.

Toilets

Toilets on coaches, like those on aircraft, are impressive more for their ingenuity in fitting everything into a small space than for their comfort and accessibility. But many people who never need to use them are nevertheless reassured because they are there. All Caledonian and National Express London-Scotland services are advertised to have toilets; Scottish Citylink says that all its Cordon Bleu services are equipped and other coaches on London-Scotland routes 'are normally fitted with toilet/ washroom'.

But Citylink's services within Scotland, and a considerable part of National Express's network, are serviced by coaches without toilets. National has introduced a new type of coach, fitted with a toilet as standard, and these will gradually be used on more and more routes, but at present, only Rapides and Anglo-Scottish services guarantee it.

Some coach journeys involve a change of vehicle. There are important coach interchanges at Birmingham, Leeds, Bristol, Cambridge, Leicester, Manchester, Nottingham, Preston, Sheffield, Edinburgh and Glasgow, where arrivals and departures are arranged to give adequate time for people to change vehicles and transfer their luggage. Many people interchange at London's Victoria Coach Station too.

There are coach services linking airports (such as Gatwick, Heathrow and Luton) with each other and with many parts of the country direct, enabling people to avoid the expense of taking a car to the airport when going on holiday.

Not all passengers start and finish their coach travel at coach stations. There are many pick-up points on the way, some no more than a bus stop in a village street. If you are boarding a coach at such a point, make sure of the time when it is due, be at the stop in good time and make sure you are on the right side of the road. Stand in a position where the driver will be able to see you, especially at night.

Holidays by coach

Coach holidays designed with older people in mind have been a staple of the coach industry for many years: they are very popular, and the coach operator is always keen to get it right precisely because you are such an important source of trade. Talk with someone who is familiar with local coach firms and find out who offers the best service.

Besides the express services, coaches also provide holiday travel (including the European mainland) and a whole range of sightseeing and excursion trips. Some of these, days out to stately homes or sporting events, are advertised by coach companies and open to all who want to book in advance. But coach companies also provide group travel for clubs, churches and societies of all kinds.

Many coach companies will provide programmes of suggested excursions for club secretaries. There is even a monthly magazine, *Group Travel Organiser,* giving details of places to visit and how to get there. Club travel organising secretaries can apply to be included in its free circulation by ringing 071-735 5058.

Accessible coaching

Coaches are not generally very accessible for people with disabilities. Most coaches have the floor at a higher level than buses. This is to allow space for luggage lockers underneath, but it means that there are several steps to climb, which are steep and high. Some of the newer coaches such as the National Express 'Expressliners' have a 'kneeling facility': this means that at a touch of a switch the driver can lower the coach on its springs to bring the bottom step nearer to the ground. Other coaches have an extra bottom step which slides into place to help people board.

There are a limited number of coaches with lifts for wheelchair users and your local coach company will give you details. National Express will carry wheelchair users provided that they can transfer to a standard coach seat and that the wheelchair is collapsible and can be stowed in the luggage locker. A phone call to the nearest National Express or Caledonian Express Office at least seven days before the journey will ensure that 'customer care' staff make arrangements to help a disabled passenger. The Bus and Coach Council (see p 153) publish a booklet listing bus and coach operators who have lift-equipped vehicles.

'Ride the motorway, catch a glimpse of the by-way' may be a more appropriate coaching slogan for today. But coaching has come a long way since the first daily, year-round service was started between Bristol and London in 1925, and it offers an inexpensive way of travelling for those whose schedules are not too demanding.

COMMUNITY TRANSPORT
John Taylor

Despite the growth in the number of low step buses, and easy to enter trains, many people still find using public transport difficult. It is estimated that somewhere between 7 per cent and 12 per cent of the population either cannot use public transport, or find it a problem.

Many of these people do not have a car of their own, and most of them are older people.

This has led to a growth in alternative transport schemes run by non-profit making bodies which are collectively known as 'community transport'. Community transport is difficult to define, but if you think of it as transport which reaches the people other transport does not reach, you will not go too far wrong. There is a variety of services, some aimed at individual travellers, and some aimed at groups of people travelling together.

Social car schemes

Social car schemes involve a central organisation recruiting and co-ordinating a local pool of drivers who are happy to give other people lifts, in return for expenses. Many different organisations run car schemes, including Age Concern (see p 157), the Women's Royal Voluntary Service (WRVS) (see p 154), the Red Cross (see p 153) and local community councils. The size and style of scheme will vary from area to area depending upon local needs and resources. In some areas, the schemes are very small, but Shropshire, for example, is covered by a network of 70 schemes, with 1,000 drivers undertaking half a million miles each year, and taking up 10 per cent of the county council's public transport budget.

Most schemes concentrate on meeting the mobility needs of older or disabled people, and usually there are some restrictions on the types and lengths of journeys which can be undertaken. A non-profit fare or contribution to costs will be expected. Usually, the cost works out as being more expensive than a bus, but cheaper than a taxi.

Dial-a-rides

Dial-a-rides offer a door-to-door transport service using minibuses or light vans adapted with fold out steps, extra handrails, and passenger lifts so that they are easy to get in and out of, and can even accommodate passengers in wheelchairs. They are to be found in all the metropolitan areas, and most major towns, under a number of different names, including:

- Dial-a-Ride: London, South Yorkshire, Hampshire, Nottinghamshire, Cheshire
- Dial-a-Bus: Derby, Strathclyde
- Ring & Ride: Greater Manchester, West Midlands, Cleveland
- Merseylink: Merseyside
- Carecall: Tyne and Wear
- Access Bus: West Yorkshire
- Readibus: Reading
- Handicabs: Lothian
- Freedom Travel: Fylde Coast

It is important to understand that although most of these are run by not-for-profit organisations, there is nothing charitable about them. They are simply 'bus' services for people unable to use the ordinary bus.

You telephone to book in advance, and they will pick you up at your home and take you to your destination. They are usually only available to people who live in the local area.

The type of service differs from place to place: some will take you anywhere within their operating area, whereas others concentrate on a few selected destinations such as the shopping centre, the health centre, and the railway station. The size of area within which they operate may vary. A few will take you on long distance journeys, but most are limited to local journeys only. Fares will be charged, but it may be possible to use your concessionary pass or tokens. The number of trips you can book at once, and the length of time in advance you are allowed to book differ from scheme to scheme. Some schemes will not take people to hospital for treatment as they do not wish to usurp the functions of the ambulance service.

The rapidly increasing demand for this sort of service has surprised most politicians and planners, and no scheme yet has enough vehicles to meet all the requests for transport which it receives. Dial-a-rides are more likely to be able to accommodate your request if you are flexible as to the time when you want to travel, so that they can fit you in with the needs of other travellers.

Most dial-a-rides will want you to register with them in advance. The sort of questions they will ask to start with are:

Are you able to use public transport? If not why not? Some people may have a medical problem which comes and goes, so that they can use a bus on some days, but not on others. They would be expected to use the bus if they can, but use the dial-a-ride when they need to.

Where do you live? (Only local residents are eligible.)

This will decide whether you are eligible. A typical dial-a-ride then asks the following questions:

What difficulty do you have with public transport?

What is the nature of your mobility problem? (These two questions are for research purposes and will help plan new services. But it can also help the drivers if they know in advance that, for example, you are partially sighted.)

Name, address and telephone number. Where is the entrance to your home?

What mobility aids do you use (wheelchair, walking stick, walking frame, etc.)

Age.

Whether you are a concessionary pass holder.

Name and phone number of a third party to contact in case they cannot get in touch with you (family or a friend or neighbour).

Any destinations you will want to go to regularly (most

dial-a-rides keep their information on computer, and having this information in advance saves them precious time).

They will then give you a membership number. When the time comes to book a trip, they will want to know:

- your name and membership number
- where you want to be picked up from
- when you want to be picked up
- where you want to go to
- whether you are travelling alone or with a companion
- whether you have an appointment for a particular time (i.e. whether you can be flexible in your timing)
- whether you want to book a return trip, and if so when

Women's Safe Transport

In our large towns, many women do not go out at night because they are afraid of being attacked. This is partly due to a loss of confidence in the public transport system during the hours of darkness. As a result, there has been a growth in special transport systems run in the evenings by women, for women. Usually called Women's Safe Transport schemes, there were by the end of 1989 about a dozen in operation in London, Bristol, Bradford, and other large towns. They usually operate on the dial-a-ride principle and take you from door to door. Older women make quite a lot of use of these schemes.

Community minibuses

In many areas, voluntary organisations such as Age Concern or community councils have found that the only way to bring people in to their meetings is to operate their own minibuses and pick their members up and take them home. A large number of these minibuses are adapted to make them easy and safe for people who have difficulty getting into ordinary buses. They serve luncheon clubs, day centres, friendship groups and so on, and are also used for outings.

It isn't always economic for a single group to own its own minibus, so increasingly a special organisation is set up just to run minibuses for other voluntary organisations. These are often called Community Transport Groups. They do not usually put on transport for individuals, unless they are operating a dial-a-ride as well. However, a group of older people getting together to go on an outing should be able to hire a suitable minibus from them quite cheaply, and they may well be able to organise a volunteer to drive.

Increasingly, these minibuses are fitted with seat belts on every seat. These are there for your safety and comfort. If you are a wheelchair user and can transfer from your wheelchair into a seat, do so. It is safer, and will leave more room for other people in the vehicle. If you do stay in your wheelchair, then ensure that not only is it clamped down firmly, but also that you are given at least a lap belt to use.

Longer journeys

If you want to undertake a longer journey and need a special transport service, it may be possible for you to be taken by your local dial-a-ride group to the railway station, and picked up by another dial-a-ride at the station at the other end. To plan this sort of journey, contact your local dial-a-ride group first. If you are going abroad, you will find that there are similar groups based in other countries, but reciprocal arrangements are as yet not very well developed. However, organisations such as the British Red Cross (see p 153) may also assist.

The following should be able to give you information about whether there are any of the above services in your area:

- Community Transport Association (see p 153)
- your local council for voluntary service or community council
- The public transport section in your local county or regional council or passenger transport authority
- TRIPSCOPE

FURTHER READING

- *Community Transport Magazine,* published six times a year by the Community Transport Association.

CYCLING
John Taylor

Pedal power

Cycling is the most energy efficient way of getting around. Despite all the developments of lightweight plastics and lean-burn car engines, there is nothing as effective as a pair of legs turning a pair of pedals. There is no mass cycling tradition amongst older people in the United Kingdom as, say, in Holland, where lots of senior citizens cycle to places which they would not be able to reach by foot. Nevertheless, there are many older British cyclists who will tell you of the fitness and fun they get out of their machines.

What could be more convenient for nipping down to the shops? Your bicycle saves you the trouble of walking all the way there and back, or getting the car out and having to worry about parking at the other end.

You may not have cycled for some time, but that does not matter. Cycling is a bit like swimming: once you have learnt how to do it, you may get rusty but you never forget. To get back in the swing of things, take it easy – pick a Sunday morning in a quiet area to practice, before venturing back on to the roads. One good thing has occurred in the last few years – modern tyre design means that punctures occur far less frequently than before.

Equipment

Cycling is a growing market, and manufacturers have responded with a great variety of models. There are:

- racing bicycles
- touring bicycles
- mountain bicycles
- off-road bicycles
- fold-away bicycles

- tandems
- tricycles

These are generally available in both 'ladies' and 'gents' versions, and with different frame sizes to suit your height and leg length. The important thing is to buy for 'function' rather than for 'looks', and not to worry about the latest gadgets – the basic design of bicycles has not changed for the last 80 years.

Despite the cheap offers in the papers and discount chain stores, the best place to get good personal service and sound advice is a bicycle shop. Before going, think about the types of journeys you might want to do – just local trips to do the shopping or see friends, days out in the country, or even cycling holidays, carrying your gear with you. This will help the shop recommend the sort of bicycle you might look for.

New bicycles can seem expensive. Of course, when you calculate how much you will save on the cost of running a car or taking public transport, it soon becomes clear what good value cycling is, quite apart from the fact that it is much healthier for you. However, if you cannot afford a new bicycle do not despair. Make it clear that you have a limited budget, and the shop may be able to recommend a second-hand bicycle, or even sell you one itself.

At 1990 prices, kitting yourself out might cost something like this:

A reasonably lightweight five or ten speed touring bicycle	£160
Waterproof cape	£10
Basket	£6
Luggage rack	£8
Saddlebag	£15
Lights and batteries	£12
Reflective leg bands	£5
Small tool and puncture repair kit	£3
'U' type security lock	£16
Total	**£235**

Running costs are very low. Even allowing for buying five sets of batteries and new inner tubes every year, together with occasional new tyres, having the bicycle serviced annually at a bicycle shop, Cyclists Touring Club Membership and a comprehensive 'New for Old' insurance policy, the cost over five years should not exceed £280. This means that the total cost of purchasing and running the bicycle works out at around £2.00 per week, or £1.60 per week if you take into account the fact that you can sell everything at the end of this time. Compare this figure with the weekly cost of bus or train travel, or running a car.

Before buying a bicycle, try it out. The important things, apart from obvious matters such as the general state of a second-hand bicycle, are whether it can be adjusted so that you feel comfortable getting on and off, and in the cycling position; and, secondly, whether you can achieve a natural rhythm when pedalling. We have all got this rhythm, called 'cadence', and the point of the gears is to enable us to keep pedalling at the constant speed which we find easiest, whilst the gears enable us to go slower up hills, and faster down them. By this means, we use the least energy.

The moral is, 'if you don't feel comfortable on it, don't buy it'. One way of getting more comfortable, of course, is to buy a good saddle, and here you can get good advice from the bicycle shop.

Cycling in traffic

There is no doubt that today's traffic conditions mean that cycling in major towns at certain times of the day is not enjoyable. The simple answer is: 'Don't do it'. Plan your journey so that you can avoid rush hours and congested streets. Town planners are slowly increasing the number of cycle routes and cycle lanes in our towns, and local cycling groups such as the London Cycling Campaign (see p 154) publish route maps which avoid main roads. There is a quite special pleasure to be obtained from moving down an empty cycle lane past a queue of frustrated car drivers.

Riding in traffic requires a firm knowledge of the highway code, and the special rules which apply to cyclists. Remember that you can be prosecuted for breaking certain traffic laws on a bicycle just as much as in a car. There are two philosophical approaches: the pragmatic and the forceful.

Pragmatic cyclists recognise that car drivers are dangerous lunatics in charge of hurtling lumps of steel. They dismount when they meet potentially dangerous obstacles such as roundabouts, or turning right. They do not try to squeeze through narrow gaps, but wait their turn.

Forceful cyclists, on the other hand, are confident in their own abilities. They know exactly where they are going, and make this quite clear with emphatic signals. They deliberately take up a position in the middle of their lane, to prevent cars overtaking, and they do not let themselves be intimidated by other people's driving behaviour.

Either of these strategies will work. The one to avoid is the halfway stage, whereby signals are not clearly given, and decisions to move out into traffic are made at the last second. This will lead to accidents.

Other things to consider are bright clothing, wearing reflective strips, and ensuring that all lights and reflectors on the bicycle are in good order. Carrying a lot of weight is not a good idea in heavy traffic as it often causes a cyclist to weave, particularly if it is mounted high up, or unequally distributed on one side of the bicycle. Another problem area is things catching in the wheels: do not allow this to happen, as the bicycle will stop dead and you will be catapulted over the front handlebars. Wheel-covers can help, but it all adds to the weight of your bicycle. Plastic bags hanging from the handlebars are very dangerous.

The weather

Despite the notorious reputation of the English weather, it actually does not rain that often. Nevertheless, cycling in the rain is not a very uplifting experience, and most people try to wait for the clouds to pass by. If wet weather cycling is unavoidable, make sure that you are carrying some waterproof gear. The usual key piece of clothing is a cape which covers the cyclist and the handlebars. You can get waterproof trousers as well, but unless these are made of a material that 'breathes', which is expensive, you will get as wet with them on as without, and it may be better to ensure that the clothes which you wear when cycling are of the 'dry quickly' variety.

Almost as problematic as the rain, is the sunshine. Firstly, it is quite easy to get very thirsty when cycling, so make sure you are carrying a bottle of liquid. Secondly, cyclists tend to forget that although wearing a T-shirt and shorts keeps them cool when they are out on long hot summer afternoons, it does not stop the sun's rays getting to their skin. Sun cream should be applied liberally to the parts at risk. Wearing a cap is a good idea, particularly for those who are a bit thin on top.

Cycle theft

This is becoming endemic in our major cities, both of parts of bicycles, and of whole machines. But if you are sensible, you will be unlucky if you have a problem. Here are some points to note:

Lock your bicycle at all times when you are not on it. If you keep it in a shed outside your house, lock it in there as well. Make sure it is locked to something solid, and that the lock goes round the frame and through both wheels, as well as the lamp-post, railing, road sign or whatever. If your bicycle is worth a lot of money, invest in a special hardened steel lock such as the 'Citadel'. Ordinary bicycle locks made of chain or wire rope take a determined thief between one and four seconds to sever with bolt cutters, although they will obviously prevent the casual thief.

Park your bicycle in as public place as possible, and if you can keep an eye on it when you are in the bank, doing the shopping, having a meal, do so.

Take off everything which can be removed without a spanner and take it with you. This will usually be the front and back lights and the pump. This is easy if you have a removable pannier which you can carry everything in.

When you buy your bicycle, ask the shop to security stamp it. This involves stamping a code number into the frame. If they do not undertake the service, the local police crime prevention unit will do. This will enable the police to trace you as the owner if they recover the bicycle when stolen.

Insure your bicycle, and check that the insurance covers the full amount you would have to pay to replace it.

Getting out

After you have built up confidence with local trips, you may want to become more adventurous. This is the chance for you to sit down armed with a set of Ordnance Survey maps, and a gazetteer of places to see in the area you want to explore. Plan your routes so that you can quickly get off the main roads and down the country by-ways. Seated on a bicycle you are at an ideal height for looking over most country hedges, but remember that when you look to the right, the body automatically starts to steer left. The maps will also help you avoid the steep hills.

Some people prefer cycling on their own, but if you prefer the conviviality and security which cycling in a group can give you, there is a network of cycling clubs covering the country, most of which have 'veterans' sections. Members generally meet socially every week, and go out riding together every weekend. Not all members are sinewy octogenarians warming up after 75 years in the saddle – they also plan shorter rides for those who want to take it a bit easier. Contact the Cyclists' Touring Club (see p 154) for more details of local activity.

Recently, the popularity of recreational cycling has been recognised by the creation of special cycle paths away from roads, often from disused branch railway lines which are perfect because they have such a level gradient. The Tissington Trail in the Derbyshire Peak District is a very good example. At some of these popular tourist spots, there are arrangements for bicycle hire, so you can arrive by car or public transport and pick up a bicycle locally.

The general policy of British Rail is that bicycles are carried on trains without charge, which is a great boon to cyclists. There are, however, restrictions to this, because some trains are too crowded, and modern trains may not have a guards van. On some InterCity and Express services, a reservation is necessary and a £3 charge is made. This is outlined in the leaflet: *The Rail Travellers' Guide to Biking by Train'*, available from your nearest station.

Abroad

Having met a pensioner cycling down the Karakoram Highway, a road which climbs to nearly 18,000 feet crossing the Himalayas from Pakistan to China, I am no longer surprised by what older people do abroad on two wheels. However, most of us want to be lowered gently into this sort of thing, and it is probably better to start with a cycle holiday company, which does all the organisation for you, and may even carry your luggage from hotel to hotel (or camp-site to camp-site), leaving you the joy of care-free cycling with just a few essentials, on a route as long or short as you want. A well-known and frequently recommended company which specialises in cycling holidays in France, is Susi Madron's Cycling for Softies, (see p 154). Their 'Local Laze About', or 'Gentle Tourer' holidays on easy terrain, seem particularly appropriate. Other similar companies advertise in the Sunday papers.

The Club

Whether you stay at home or go abroad, membership of the Cyclists' Touring Club (see p 154) is strongly recommended. In addition to producing a magazine, organising very economical bicycle insurance, arranging free legal aid and third party insurance for members, they also offer a leisure cycling advisory service with maps, routes, and information on where to go and how to get there. Their technical advisory service answers individual queries, but also produces information sheets on equipment selection, how best to carry luggage, and how to care for your cycle. Of particular interest is the information which they can supply on cycling for those who have a disability. This will also interest older people whose legs are no longer as strong as they used to be, as it considers the advantages of tricycles, as well as more specialist equipment.

Membership for people aged 65 or over is only £9.25 per year – a 50 per cent discount.

CASE HISTORY

Dorothy has recently retired and lives by herself in Northwich. She does not have a car, as she never learnt to drive. Two summers ago she went to stay with an old school friend in Cambridge who, along with her husband, still cycles regularly. It was good weather, so her friend arranged for Dorothy to borrow a bicycle, and after a certain amount of practice, the three of them cycled the few miles out to Grantchester. Dorothy rediscovered how easy cycling is.

When she got home, she bought a second-hand ladies bicycle with a basket on the front, which was advertised in the local Post Office for £50. She uses it two or three times a week to go shopping in fine weather, as it saves waiting for the bus. She has also been out bird-watching in Delamere Forest, about five miles away, and has used it to visit her sister in Altrincham, by taking it with her on the train, and cycling a couple of miles at the other end.

FURTHER READING

- *Richard's New Bicycle Book* by Richard Ballantine, published by Pan – a comprehensive guide to choosing and using a bicycle, price £9.99.
- *The Penguin Book of the Bike* published by Penguin price £4.95.

GOING ABROAD

Graham Lightfoot

Foreign travel was once restricted to the very wealthy, who used to despatch their sons on a grand tour of Europe to finish their education. Now, of course, travelling abroad is much more widely available, especially for older people. Furthermore, a much broader selection of countries are welcoming foreign visitors; there is so much on offer, your real difficulty will be in deciding where to start.

Planning

The main considerations when going abroad are:

- the documents required
- your health
- learning about the country or countries you are visiting
- communicating with the local inhabitants
- financial arrangements

In addition to a travel agency, two useful initial sources of information are:

The embassy, tourist office or similar establishment in the UK of the country or countries you are visiting.

The Consular Department of the Foreign and Commonwealth Office (see p 154), in London.

They give advice on circumstances or events which could affect the safety and security of British nationals travelling abroad; warn about unusual problems in countries and the effect of events, such as civil disturbances and natural disasters; and provide, on request, specific notes on countries covering subjects such as climate, health and currency.

Paperwork

Relevant documents to take with you when you are going abroad can include:

Your passport, either a full passport valid for 10 years or a Visitor's Pass valid for one year. Application forms for both can be obtained from your local Post Office. In the case of a full passport, the completed form must be sent to your Regional Passport Office (as indicated on the form) and can take up to three months to obtain; although if you are able to attend in person and willing to wait you can obtain one on the same day (arrive as early as possible). In the case of a Visitor's Pass, this can be issued to you at the Post Office immediately, but it is only valid for European Community countries, Malta, Austria and Switzerland.

Visa(s): check with the relevant embassy.

Vaccination certificate(s).

Form E111, available from the Post Office (see below).

Insurance certificate(s) for both yourself and, if you are taking it, your car (see also Part 1, Insurance in the Planning section on page 18).

Driving licence: check with the relevant embassy whether your UK licence will be valid.

Car registration document, or authorisation to drive the car.

Proxy and postal voting whilst you are away. If you are going to be abroad when there are elections at which you are entitled to vote, then contact the Electoral Registration Officer at your local district or borough council for Form RPF9, which will enable you to record a postal vote before you go or to appoint a proxy to vote on your behalf.

Language

Some form of the English language is spoken by some of the inhabitants of every country in the world. But it is always very useful, if not polite, to be able to communicate with people in their own language. Pocket guides can be of assistance, but try to learn, or at least write down, some of the words and phrases which you think will be most useful and easiest to say, such as those related to food, drink, accommodation and travel. Where there is a different alphabet, eg Greek, try learning to recognise some of these useful words on road signs and so on.

If you are able to plan your trip abroad well ahead, why not enrol in a language class at your local adult education centre? When you get to your destination, you will be able to help your companions.

The right way to go

It is always worth comparing the different ways of going abroad in order to travel in the most comfortable way for the price. One of the benefits of being an island nation is the wide range of travel options open to someone wanting to leave. Air travel may be the quickest, but there are a number of coach/sea and train/sea services which are organised for through journeys. They are often cheaper and, for centre-to-centre trips, can be just as quick, especially if a hovercraft or jetfoil crossing is available. If you are in a small group, going by car and sea can work out the cheapest per person, but this is very dependent on the time of year: the cost difference between the low and high season can be as much as 100 per cent. Your travel agent will have detailed information on all the choices open to you.

Money abroad

Most banks have details of the services available to you when travelling abroad. It is very easy nowadays to travel abroad and not have to carry large amounts of cash with you. You can make particularly wide use of credit cards to obtain cash advances, goods and services.

You can buy travellers' cheques. These should be ordered, together with foreign currency, from your local bank, and from a few building societies and travel agencies. You sign the cheques in front of the bank clerk; when you cash them abroad, you sign them again at a foreign bank, large shop or hotel, many of whom will want to see your passport or other similar identification. Remember to keep a separate record of the cheques' serial numbers, both with you and back home, in case of loss or theft.

You can take Eurocheques (with a Eurocheque Card), which are available from your bank, and unlike travellers' cheques, are debited to your account in the same way as ordinary cheques (as you use them). They can also be used to obtain cash from selected banks in certain countries outside Europe.

Look after yourself

A very useful reference booklet, available free from the Department of Health, is *The Traveller's Guide to Health: Vital Information You Should Know Before Travelling Abroad.* It provides various health check-lists, advice on vaccination for all the countries in the world, and details of emergency medical treatment in non-European countries with reciprocal health agreements with Britain.

If you are travelling in the European Community, you should carry a form known as E111. The leaflet about it *(Health Care for Visitors to E.C. Countries: How to get emergency treatment with your E111)* is available from the Post Office: simply fill the form in, at the back, and the counter staff will do the rest. They may ask you for some proof of your identity. This form makes it possible to claim back certain medical costs incurred because of urgent treatment for accident or unexpected illness. The different arrangements for each country are outlined in the leaflet.

British Airways has established a network of Travel Clinics in major cities in the UK. For an up-to-date list of these clinics telephone 071-831 5333. You will probably have to make an appointment if you wish to be seen at a specific time. They can provide advice and the latest information from the London School of Hygiene and Tropical Medicine as well as on the spot immunisation. The Travel Clinics also stock a range of items such as needle and syringe packs, mosquito nets, water purifiers and insect repellant.

Another source of information, advice and equipment is the Medical Advisory Service for Travellers Abroad (MASTA) (see p

154). MASTA can provide you with various levels of personal health briefings at a set fee depending upon which country you are visiting. MASTA application forms are available from the pharmacist at all branches of Boots the Chemist, Savory & Moore and R. Gordon Drummond or by phoning MASTA on 071-631 4408.

Frailty and disability

It is worth contacting the national and local pensioners' or disability organisations of the country or countries you are visiting, for:

- access and travel details
- assistance with any problems
- hiring, loaning or repairing of specialist equipment
- items of general interest

The contacts for disability organisations in many countries are contained in the RADAR publication *Holidays and Travel Abroad 1990/91: A Guide for Disabled People.* Age Concern England have also produced Factsheet No 4 – *Holidays For Elderly People,* which may be of use.

Problems whilst you are there

In the event of any serious problems, for example if your money or passport are stolen, or you fall ill, then try to contact British Consular officials. They can give direct assistance and advise of local procedures.

FURTHER READING

- *Holidays and Travel Abroad 1990/91: A Guide for Disabled People* published by RADAR price £3.00 inc. p & p.
- *Life in the Sun* by Nancy Tuft, published by Age Concern England, price £6.95.
- *The Traveller's Guide to Health: Vital Information You Should Know Before Travelling Abroad,* available free from the

Department of Health. Phone (free of charge) 0800 555 777; it is also updated on Prestel page 50063 (Prestel is often available in local libraries).

■ *Your Social Security, Health Care and Pension Rights in the European Community,* available free from your local department of social security office.

GRANDCHILDREN

Richard Armitage

If you have grandchildren (or other children you take care of), travel can be a great way to spend time together. Like everything else, there are a few rules to watch out for and planning always pays off.

Children in transit

Try to remember what you felt like when you went on journeys when you were a child. Children will find travel exciting and different, but you need to pay especial attention to being able to satisfy their essential needs on demand (that is, not necessarily at the next convenient stop along the way). In particular, toileting (frequent stops, nappies), food and drink (preferably consumables that create as little mess as possible), and games and entertainment (bookshops have books on games to play with children when you are travelling).

Children and cars

The new seat belt laws affect drivers and children in the back of cars. As from 1st September 1989, if seat belts or child restraints are fitted in the rear of a car, it is the driver's legal responsibility to see that children under 14 years of age use them - even if it is the first time you ever gave a child a lift. The seat belt or restraint must be appropriate for the age and weight of the child. This law is in addition to all existing legislation for car drivers and front seat passengers.

Ideally, a child should be restrained in a purpose-designed restraint appropriate to their weight (you will find the weight on the equipment's label). For children under one year old, a carrycot which is itself restrained by straps or an infant carrier; for children one to three years old, a child seat, harness or booster cushion used in conjunction with an adult seat belt; four to fourteen years old, the adult belt. Some local authority road safety sections and some health authorities are now lending out child car safety equipment at little or no cost, so you may not need to buy any additional equipment outright. Further information is available from the Department of Transport on Freephone 0800 234888.

Concessions

Many forms of transport (buses, coaches, trains, planes, and ferries) offer concessions for children travelling accompanied by an adult; in some cases, very young children travel free. Remember this, next time you are organising a journey: perhaps a child could go with you too?

HOSPITAL

John Taylor

Some people without cars find particular difficulty getting to hospital. This problem is likely to get worse as small local hospitals continue to be closed down, and modern hospitals are built at the edge of towns, rather than in the centre. Below are some of the ways these problems can be overcome.

Check with your doctor whether you are eligible for an ambulance. An ambulance should be provided for those receiving treatment who are considered by a doctor to be 'medically unfit to travel by other means'. If the doctor considers that you should have an ambulance, they will arrange it. In some areas this will be a proper ambulance, in others a minibus, whilst in others it may be a car.

Telephone the hospital, or the local bus information line, for details of the bus service to the hospital. Councils responsible for planning the bus services make a particular effort to provide a service to hospitals, and often print special leaflets about them.

Many hospitals organise a 'Hospital Car Service' using volunteers who are happy to give lifts to people with difficulties using public transport. This may be because they cannot get on or off the buses, or because there is no bus which runs in the right place at the right time. You will be expected to pay something towards this service, but it will be cheaper than a taxi.

If you are no longer able to use buses, and there is a dial-a-ride in your area, it will take you to hospital, but generally only as a visitor. Most dial-a-rides will not take people to hospitals for treatment, as they feel that this is a job for the ambulance service. If you have difficulty in getting to hospital for treatment, give the dial-a-ride a ring to discuss the problem with them.

Find out from your local council for voluntary service or Citizens Advice Bureau whether there is a voluntary car scheme or other community transport scheme covering your area.

You may be able to get help from the hospital with your travel costs. You are entitled to help if:

You or your partner receive Income Support or Family Credit.

You are being treated for the disability for which you get a War or MOD Disablement Pension.

You live in the area covered by the Highlands & Islands Development Board in Scotland and have to travel at least 30 miles (or more than five miles by water) to get to hospital.

You live in the Isles of Scilly and have to travel to the mainland.

You are on a low income.

Generally you have to be receiving treatment to get a refund of the money you spend on fares (including taxi fares if there is no other way you can travel). However, if you are accompanying someone who needs assistance, then you should both claim. Take your Income Support or Family Credit Order Book, or letters about benefit, to the hospital general office and show them to a member of staff there. They will then organise a refund for you, if you are eligible.

Usually, refunds are made at the hospital each time you visit. If you are not going back to the hospital, the refund will be forwarded by post. If you are on a low income you will not receive money straight away from the hospital. You must ask for form AG1 from the hospital general office, complete it and post it back. If you do not have enough money to get to the hospital, ask them to send you payment in advance, or apply to your local social security office. If you want to visit someone, but cannot afford the fares, you may be able to get help from the Social Fund, available through your local social security office. Full details are contained in the Department of Health leaflet 'H11', available at the social security office, and the hospital.

LONDON

Ian Yearsley

Travel in London is full of conflicting experiences: on the one hand there are all the tourist sites and on the other there can be severe congestion. These experiences highlight several important points about travel through London:

London is one of the world's most fascinating cities, and is extensively provided with public transport.

The transport network has become grossly overloaded and congested in recent years; numbers using the Underground have risen by 70 per cent since 1982. Buses, though not so crowded, are subject to delays caused by traffic congestion.

There is an enormous amount of information available, if you know where to get it.

This section, therefore, looks first at ways of avoiding having to cross London (if you are on your way to somewhere else), then at ways of reducing the aggravation if you need to cross London, and finally the travel opportunities within London.

Even for those who know the capital well, crossing London can be tricky.

CASE HISTORY

Mrs. Aldridge who lives in Kent wants to visit her sister in Sheffield but puts it off because she cannot face the crush of people in the Underground trains, whilst crossing between mainline rail stations in London.

Mrs. Aldridge's problem of a journey from Kent to Sheffield can be solved, not by a through train, but by using British Rail's Thameslink which connects Brighton, Gatwick, East Croydon and other places south of London with Luton and Bedford. If she travels to London Bridge station, from the same platform or one nearby every half hour there will be a Thameslink train, burrowing under the city in its own tunnel and out to Luton or Bedford, where she can join for Sheffield. No overcrowding like the Underground, and there's even a buffet trolley to serve a cup of tea. Mrs. Aldridge should check the timings before she sets out, to make sure everything connects as smoothly as possible. She would find it a good idea to reserve a seat on the Sheffield train as well as the train into London Bridge.

Mr. Birtwistle in Croydon is reluctant to accept his daughter's invitation for a holiday in Manchester, because he cannot cope with crowded escalators on the Victoria Line.

If London is not your destination, why not avoid it altogether? Mr. Birtwistle in Croydon, who wants to avoid escalators, could use one of the through trains from Brighton or Eastbourne to Manchester which call at East Croydon and avoid the centre of London by going via Clapham Junction and Kensington Olympia.

Folkestone, Dover and Gatwick Airport all have through trains to Midlands and Northern destinations, and there are trains from Edinburgh and Glasgow to Brighton.

In general the overall journey time is longer by these trains than by using the ordinary services in and out of London and braving the London crossing. But if you are not in a hurry and prefer to use a more relaxing through train, they are worth thinking about.

There are also some Midlands to South services via Reading instead of London, and further afield there are 'Express' services from Harwich and East Anglia to Liverpool and Blackpool, and InterCity trains from the North East to the West Country.

National Express (see p 153) and other coach operators now provide services to destinations north or south of London, using the M25 motorway to avoid the congested central area.

Crossing London

If none of the through services fits your needs, you will want to look at ways of reducing the aggravation of crossing London. The railway map of Britain looks rather like a spider's web, with lines converging on London. A journey from Oxford to Cambridge, for instance, almost certainly means going round two sides of a triangle via London, with the long Underground or taxi journey from Paddington to King's Cross or Liverpool Street in the middle.

Through tickets

British Rail through tickets nowadays normally include the cross-London Underground fare and they have chocolate- coloured magnetic stripes on the back to work the Underground's automatic ticket gates. On most tickets there is a + symbol next to the destination to show that the cross-London fare is included.

Avoiding the peaks

Try to time your journey to avoid arriving in London during the evening peak period (which means any time from 4 pm to 7.30 pm) and the morning peak (7.30 am to 10.00 am). Sunday evenings can also be very busy.

London Underground

On London's Underground there is a zone fare system. All its stations serving British Rail InterCity terminals (except Kensington Olympia) are in Zone 1, and (at the time of writing) the fare between them is 70p. You can get your ticket from the automatic machine set in the wall or the ticket office. Some machines (simply) offer a range of prices, but usually there is at least one with a button for each destination. Usually these machines give change, but sometimes they run out , so have a supply of 10p, 20p, 50p and £1 coins ready.

Automatic barriers

Whether you buy a ticket from a machine, ticket office or use a British Rail through ticket, you will need to insert it into an automatic barrier gate. Place it into the slot nearest to you on the right hand side of the barrier, with the brown stripe downwards. It will reappear from another slot nearer the barrier, and the display will light up 'Take Ticket'. Only when you retrieve your ticket from the slot will the barrier open and the display change to 'Enter'. If there is a problem with your ticket 'seek assistance' will light up. There should be a station guard nearby to help you sort out the problem. Push your luggage through in front of you, otherwise the barrier may close behind you leaving your luggage stranded outside. There is a door at the end of each set of automatic ticket barriers which can be opened for you, if for example you have a lot of luggage. When you leave the Underground, the procedure is just the same at the exit barrier.

London's buses

London has a vast network of bus services, all controlled by London Transport (see p 155). But not all buses belong to London Buses or are painted in the traditional red colour. Many are now provided by other companies under contract to London Transport.

This means that there are many different colours and many different types of vehicle. Some 300 of the newest buses have features such as low steps, textured handrails, bus stopping signs and large bell pushes to help those with mobility difficulties. But there are some minibuses and older double and single deck buses with varying ease of access. There are also still many routes in the central area served by traditional open rear platform buses with a conductor as well as driver. Though the steps on these may be high, at least there is someone to help you and you don't have to fumble with change to pay a fare at the same time as getting on. One legacy of the former Greater London Council is that very many of London's bus stops are provided with shelters. Most stops have some timetable information on display, though sometimes this is vandalised.

Information about bus routes and timetables can be obtained from London Transport's Travel Information Service (see p 155).

Cheap travel in London

There is a good system of Travelcards which are valid on British Rail suburban lines as well as Underground and bus services. These can be bought at British Rail Network South East Stations, Underground Stations, London Transport information offices, London Buses' garages and some newsagents but not on the buses themselves. They last for one day or longer, and besides being good value for money, save you a lot of time and searching for change every time you want to make a journey.

Taxis *see section on Taxis page 128*

At busy times you may have to queue at stations like Waterloo, Euston or Victoria, so you will need to allow extra time in your itinerary.

Riverbuses

Newly-established riverbus services may be of interest, simply for pleasure or for getting you across London. The Riverbus company (see p 155) operates an hourly service from Chelsea Harbour to Charing Cross, and a service every 20 minutes from Charing Cross to Greenwich. In addition, London City Airport (see p 154) based at King George V Dock, have their own hourly service to Charing Cross. The journey takes 35 minutes.

Watch your luggage

One warning: always keep your luggage with you and in sight at all times when crossing London. There are thieves whose speciality is to pick up luggage while the owners are looking elsewhere, buying a newspaper, asking for directions or being distracted in some way. You are especially vulnerable when you are making a call from a payphone.

Frailty and disability

The Underground is not generally wheelchair accessible, though improvements are promised for future Underground lines. For someone with walking difficulties, time should be allowed at those stations with long corridors and sets of stairs. You can find out about stations from London Transport (see p 155). Each station has a ticket office, often equipped with induction loops for the hard of hearing. The new Docklands Light Railway is fully accessible to wheelchair users, with lifts at all stations.

Carelink and other accessible buses

For the passenger with limited mobility, London Transport operate the wheelchair accessible Carelink bus service, every hour on a circular route linking Euston, St. Pancras/King's Cross, Liverpool Street, Waterloo, Victoria and Paddington. There are spaces for wheelchairs and seats for companions on this bus. Adult fare is £1, or 50p for children aged five to fifteen, for holders of British Rail Disabled Person's Railcards or London boroughs' Elderly or Disabled Person's Travel Permits.

The Carelink bus also connects with the wheelchair accessible Airbus service between central London and all four terminals at Heathrow Airport.

Disabled Passengers' Unit

London Transport have a special Unit for Disabled Passengers which provides information and services. London Transport have single deck, side lift-equipped mobility buses in several areas, and administer the London Taxicard scheme which enables severely disabled London residents to use black taxis at much reduced fares (see Taxis section on page 134).

The Unit also has large print versions of the Underground and central area bus maps. As well as a whole variety of free information leaflets, it provides a 74-page *Access to the Underground* handbook for £1 post paid or 70p over the counter at London Transport information desks. There is a shortened Braille version free of charge, and the Unit is preparing a tactile Central Area Underground Map.

As well as travel information, the Unit can also give details of lift-equipped sightseeing buses. London Transport's own museum, at Covent Garden, is fully accessible.

FURTHER READING

- *Access to the Underground* handbook, published by London Transport.

MOBILITY AIDS

John Taylor

If you find that as you get older you are beginning to have difficulty in walking, this does not mean that you have to stop going out altogether. Apart from any treatment, or special exercises, there are various technical aids available to assist your local mobility. Your starting point for information and assistance will usually be your doctor.

Sticks

The simplest aid is a walking stick, which can be obtained on prescription through your doctor, borrowed from your local social services department, or purchased from an outdoor pursuits shop. It is important that your walking stick is the correct length. It should be level with your wrist when your arm is held by your side. If you use two walking sticks, these should be longer, as they will be used more in front of you, rather than to give support to one side. The stick should be fitted with a non-slip rubber end, called a ferrule. Check this regularly as it quickly wears out. A more expensive type of walking stick, called a 'flipstick' has a fold-down seat as part of the handle. Another version of this, a 'shooting stick', has a pointed end to stick in the ground. This is useful to give you a rest when watching an outdoors event where you have to stand up. These are available from country clothing and riding equipment shops.

Frames

Walking frames give you more support and stability, and are available on prescription. Your doctor will refer you to your local hospital's physiotherapy department, who will advise you on which type you should use, and teach you how to use it.

Wheelchairs

If, on occasions, you are unable to walk even with the help of a stick or a frame, then you may need a wheelchair. There are many different types of chair, and, as with a walking frame, your doctor will arrange for professional advice for you. The wheelchair will be provided free and you can ask to be taught how to use it. However, electric wheelchairs for use outdoors are only available from the Health Service if you cannot propel a manual wheelchair and the person accompanying you cannot manage to push you. If you have the resources, you can purchase one privately. Before choosing a particular chair, ask yourself:

Am I comfortable in this chair? (They come in all different widths, lengths, heights, shapes and sizes.)

Am I strong enough to propel this chair? If not, is my companion strong enough to propel me as far as we may want to go?

Will the chair go through all the doors where I would use it, at home for example?

Will I be able to carry shopping safely and comfortably?

If I travel in a car, will the person with me be able to fold the chair up easily and store it in the car?

Pavement vehicles

If you just find it a bit tiring to get out to the shops, but don't need a stick or a wheelchair, then a 'pavement vehicle' may be the answer for you. These are sometimes called 'scooters', 'personal vehicles' or 'buggies', and some are used on roads. Costing upwards of £1,500, they are usually powered by electric batteries, and you should be able to travel up to 15 miles on a single charge. Recent regulations allow some vehicles to go at speeds of 8 m.p.h. on the road. They can carry more shopping than conventional wheelchairs, and should be manoeuvrable enough to negotiate supermarkets and other shops. The majority have a 'kerb-climbing' facility. Some can be dismantled and carried in a car boot. However, if you take one onto a wheelchair accessible bus or minibus, you should always transfer to a proper seat for the duration of the journey, as they are not as stable as conventional wheelchairs. Disconnect the battery for the duration of the journey. Although you do not need a driving licence for these vehicles, you must understand the Highway Code before you take one on the road.

Buy or hire

If you are in receipt of Mobility Allowance, or War Pensioners Mobility Supplement, you can put that towards the Motability hire purchase scheme to pay for a powered wheelchair or pavement vehicle. There are a number of companies which will hire both manual and powered wheelchairs out on a short term basis – look in Yellow Pages under 'Disabled – Vehicles and Eqpt.'. If you purchase or hire for your personal use, and you have a disability, you should be able to obtain exemption from VAT. Ask your supplier for the relevant form, or get a leaflet (701/7/86: *Aids for Handicapped Persons*), from H. M. Customs & Excise (see p 155). A final point: don't forget to insure your wheelchair.

Take good advice

Take independent advice before buying a wheelchair or a pavement vehicle from a private supplier. A number of companies specialise in this field, and you should be able to borrow wheelchairs to try out before committing yourself. It is particularly important to find out what happens if something goes wrong with the chair. Banstead Place Mobility Centre (see p 155) produces an excellent leaflet: *How to Choose a Pavement Vehicle,* which they will send you on receipt of your large stamped addressed envelope. RADAR (see p 150) produce a comprehensive book: *Wheelchairs: A Guide to Choosing a Wheelchair.* The Disabled Living Foundation (see p 155) also publishes lists of different walking aids and wheelchairs, including the names and addresses of suppliers and hire companies.

Shopmobility

As shopping centres get larger and larger, they are starting to set up what are called 'Shopmobility' schemes (over 20 running so far, in towns such as Bradford, Peterborough and Redditch). These provide a stock of wheelchairs and scooters which people with walking difficulties can borrow to do their shopping. The schemes are generally situated close to a reserved parking area, and are usually free, although a deposit may be required. At peak times, pre-booking is essential.

FURTHER READING

■ *Wheelchairs: A Guide to Choosing a Wheelchair,* £3, published by RADAR, price £3.00.

MOPEDS, SCOOTERS AND MOTORCYCLES

John Taylor

Many older people use mopeds or scooters – a less strenuous form of two-wheeled travel than a bicycle. For people who have cycled before, these are quite easy to learn to ride. Mopeds are powered two-wheelers with a maximum speed of 30 m.p.h. and a maximum engine capacity of 50cc. Anything which goes faster, or with a larger engine, is described as a motorcycle.

Licences

Anyone with an existing car driving licence which includes Group E (most do) can drive a moped – no test is needed. This licence also acts as a provisional licence for motorcycles up to 125cc engine size – 'L' plates must be carried, and pillion passengers are not allowed unless they are full motorcycle licence holders. When a full car driving licence is used as a provisional licence in this way, it is not compulsory to take the riding test – you can carry on riding with 'L' plates for as long as you like. Nevertheless, going through some training and taking the test is recommended.

If you don't have a current driving licence you can obtain a provisional licence for mopeds or motorcycles up to 125cc engine size, provided you meet the usual medical and sight requirements. This will be valid for two years only, after which you must wait for a year before you can obtain another one. So you need to pass your test before your two years are up.

Driving test and licence arrangements are currently undergoing reorganisation as part of the British attempts to harmonise our system with the rest of Europe. Amongst other things, a new basic moped and motorcycle training package is to be introduced which will mean that provisional licence holders must have attended a course of training held away from public roads before they are allowed to ride on the road.

Cheaper than cars

Mopeds and scooters are substantially cheaper to purchase and operate than cars, and can provide an individual with equivalent levels of local mobility. Approximate costs, at 1990 prices, are:

The most popular model of moped	£965
Helmet	£25
Leather gloves	£15
Waterproof and windproof jacket	£20
Nylon overtrousers	£10
Total	**£1035**

Running costs are quite cheap as mopeds return over 100 miles to the gallon. In addition, you do not need a garage or a drive to park it on. Assuming 1,500 miles a year (30 miles a week), fully comprehensive insurance, an annual service and MOT (after the first three years), the cost over five years would be £500. This means that the total cost of purchasing and running the moped works out at £5.90 per week, or £4.95 per week if you take into account the value of the moped at the end of the five years. This is about one fifth of the equivalent cost of running a car.

CASE HISTORY

Reg and his wife Ann live just outside a market town in Nottinghamshire. He plays golf two or three times a week, and is a member of his local golf club which is about five miles away. He and Ann both have driving licences, but they only have one car, and Ann needs this when she travels into town to attend an afternoon painting class, and to visit an aunt who is housebound. They did consider buying a second car, but decided that a moped would be much cheaper and would do just as well. Reg leaves his clubs in a locker at the golf course, and carries waterproof golfing clothes. He now finds that because it is so cheap to run and easy to park, he uses it instead of the car for local shopping, picking up the Sunday paper and going to the Post Office.

PETS
John Taylor

Many older people enjoy the company of pets. Having a pet does not mean that you are prevented from travelling, but obviously, there are a number of things to consider.

If it is a smaller animal such as a bird or fish or cat, it may be possible for a friend or neighbour to call in and feed it while you are away, or to look after it in their own home. It is best to leave written instructions with them as to the amount and frequency of feeding, and to tell them which vet the pet is registered with, and under what name.

You may feel happier putting a dog or cat into a local kennels or cattery, particularly if you are going away for a longer period. You will find telephone numbers for these in the local Yellow Pages, or your vet may know of one they can recommend. It is worth ringing one or two to compare prices, as they can vary quite a lot.

Holiday provisions

Many people take their dogs with them on holiday, but not usually their cats, as these prefer to stay in a territory which they are used to. You will need to ensure that the hotel or guest house where you will be staying is willing to have dogs, and find out what arrangements they make regarding the dog's sleeping and feeding. You will normally want to take a couple of bowls and the dog's blanket with you. If you cannot find somewhere to stay which will accept your dog, you could board the pet at kennels nearby to the hotel, taking it out every day, and leaving it in the kennels at night.

If you want to take your dog from the United Kingdom into the Republic of Ireland, it must be over six months old and be up to date with its inoculations. You can, however, take your dog to the Channel Islands without any restrictions, and this would be the nearest you could get to taking it 'abroad' without running into quarantine regulations.

Travelling to other countries with animals is not advisable, as on your return they will have to go into quarantine, to prevent the spread of rabies into Great Britain. This involves them spending six months in specific animal care institutions and is very costly.

Comfort

Whichever mode of travel you use, do remember that it is better for the animal if there are breaks in the journey every few hours, so that 'accidents' can be prevented. Animals can get dehydrated very easily, so it is a good idea to carry a plastic bottle of water and a small bowl with you so that the animal can have a drink. If you are carrying your pet in a box, do ensure that there is adequate ventilation, and don't make the common mistake of putting a large cushion at the bottom of the box, as this just reduces the amount of room the animal has to manoeuvre in. An old cardigan on a layer of folded newspaper is adequate.

Trains

On trains, small dogs can travel with you in the passenger compartment. Larger dogs, however, have to travel in the guard's van, and be muzzled. Other animals can be taken, provided they are in a box or basket. Theoretically, they should travel in the guard's van, for reasons of hygiene, but this is seldom enforced. The charge for taking a dog on the train is usually half fare, but subject to a maximum of £4 for a single journey and £8 for a return. Guide dogs travel free of charge.

Buses

Whether your dog is accepted on a bus is at the discretion of the driver. They may insist that you take the dog onto the top deck of a double-deck bus. They may refuse to let you on if there is already a dog on the bus, and they are worried about a possible canine conflict of opinion. However, guide dogs will only be refused if there is at least one dog already on board a small bus, or two dogs on a large single-deck or double-deck bus.

Coaches

Travelling by coach is usually slightly more restrictive. Small animals which can be confined in boxes or baskets and small dogs will be accepted, providing that the coach does not serve food or drink, as is increasingly the case with longer distance services, such as the National Express Rapide services. Larger dogs will usually not be accommodated at all, unless they are guide dogs. National Express make a charge of £1 for a single fare for a dog.

London Underground

When using the London Underground, smaller animals are not a problem, as long as they are well behaved. However, dogs are not allowed to stand on the escalators, so they have to be carried, or taken up the stairs. Some of the stations have no alternative to escalators, so this could be a problem for larger dogs. It is worth checking with the station first. The general enquiry number for the Underground is 071-222 1234. There is no charge for the animal.

Air travel

If you are flying, you will find that airlines all seem to make different arrangements. Some will only take animals as cargo, although others will take them in the passenger cabin. You will most probably have to provide an IATA approved box for them to travel in, which you can get from a vet. You will be charged for the transport of the animal, most probably at the excess baggage rate for the flight. Check the details with your travel agent before you book your ticket. On internal flights, guide dogs would normally travel in the cabin with their owner.

SEA TRAVEL
Graham Lightfoot

With the advent of the plane, it sometimes seems as though travel by boat has been forgotten. Yet, if you are going to some of the Scottish Islands, boat is actually the only way to get there. Sea travel, despite being one of the oldest forms of transport, still has much to offer the traveller and can give you a very pleasurable journey.

Planning

Details of cruises, ferries and hovercraft are all available from your local travel agent and you can then deal directly with the operator or through your travel agent. The published brochures are very detailed, but it is also worth obtaining *Access at the Channel Ports,* which includes details of port and boat facilities as well as information on shipping companies operating out of the UK.

Cost

Assuming that you are not going on a cruise nor on an organised holiday, the main points to consider include:

The availability of reductions for Senior Citizens; Scandinavian Seaways (see p 156) for example, offer a 'Senior Citizen Saver' for people travelling without a car on certain days on its sailings from Harwich.

Fares on ferries vary dramatically between different times of the year, with the most expensive fares (Summer peak) often being 60 per cent more than the cheapest fares (the depths of Winter).

On some routes there are special fares depending on the number of days between outward and return journeys, and whether you are travelling at night or by day, mid-week or week-ends.

If you are not travelling by car, then it may be cheaper to purchase your ferry ticket at the same time as your train or coach ticket; such combined tickets are usually better value than the component parts purchased separately.

The return fares are usually determined by the outward date of departure.

If you are travelling around the Western Isles of Scotland, then Caledonian MacBrayne (see p 155) offer unlimited travel tickets for a set number of days, which can be bought in advance.

Taking an overnight sailing can save on accommodation costs.

Joining Sealink British Ferries Auto Club (see p 156). This enables you to apply, after each journey, for a voucher equivalent to 20 per cent of the fare you have paid (standard fares only), which you can then use to offset the cost of future journeys.

Members of disabled motorists' organisations may travel free or at a substantial discount.

Choosing the right way to go

The main points to consider include:

Would you prefer longer land journeys and shorter sea crossings (there may be more of the latter)?

Would you prefer quicker sea crossings (hovercraft and jetfoil), which may be subject to cancellation because of rough weather, or the ferry, which will sail in these conditions?

The times of crossings, which will affect your land journeys at either end. For example: if you are driving, do you prefer to drive at night or during the day-time? If you are using public transport, arriving very early in the morning or late at night, will you have a long wait for the first bus, coach or train?

Staying overnight at the port in order to catch the early morning ferry.

If you are taking a car, for example, to Spain: do you cross Dover-Calais and then drive; or do you cross Plymouth – Santander, thus landing in Spain?

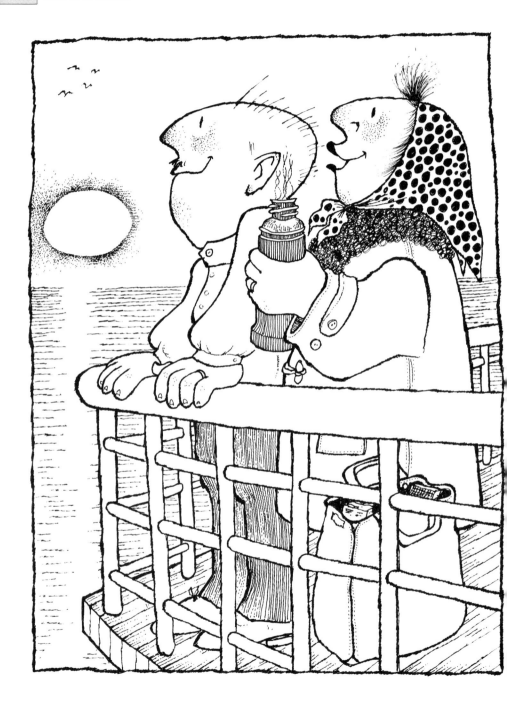

Making a booking

In most cases it is essential to book in advance, though for most ferry crossings outside the summer peak or mid-week you can just turn up at the port. It is worth checking with the ferry company in advance, especially if you have a high roof vehicle such as a motor caravan or are towing a caravan, as there are a limited number of spaces for these on each sailing.

If you are travelling by car, then you must remember to state how many passengers will be travelling; passengers not notified at the time of booking are charged extra.

Luggage

Although there are not usually any weight restrictions, some companies do have a free baggage allowance. For example, on Scandinavian Seaways (see p 156) this is 50 kilos (110 lbs) per person.

If you are travelling by car, remember to take out of the car any items which you might require during the crossing as you will not be allowed on the car deck while at sea.

Look after yourself

Always take some form of weather-proof coat and warmer clothing, especially if you intend to 'take the sea air' and go on deck.

Seasickness, even in calm seas, can pose a problem. There are various proprietary drugs available (consult your pharmacist or doctor), and your local wholefood shop should be able to recommend homoeopathic remedies which you can take. In addition, booking a cabin or just finding somewhere quiet to sit or lie down can prevent the more violent manifestations of seasickness.

Frailty and disability

If you have a disability, and in particular if you are a wheelchair user, it is essential that you book well in advance and notify the shipping company of your requirements.

Most ports and ships have lifts and most ships have a limited number of cabins which are designed to cater for wheelchair users. Hovercraft are more of a problem and you will need assistance from the car deck and will probably be asked to transfer to a seat for the crossing.

Most ships on most routes have toilets accessible to wheelchair users, but it is important to check this before booking.

Concessions are available to disabled drivers on the sailings of a number of shipping companies. In some cases this means that your car is carried free of charge or at a minimal charge to cover administrative costs.

However, most of the operators give such concessions only to members of recognised clubs such as the Disabled Drivers' Association (DDA) (see p 156) or Disabled Drivers' Motoring Club (DDMC) (see p 156). Sealink (see p 156) and B&I Line (see p 155) also give the same concessions to disabled drivers who are not members of the DDA or DDMC but they require you to complete and return a form to them.

The form must be signed by the director of your local social services or social work department certifying that you are a severely disabled driver.

Last minute hitches

Although the shipping company brochure states that there is a latest reporting time for all motorists, it is still possible to catch a ferry within a few minutes of departure time.

On some ferry routes, the service is scheduled to link with a train service or so-called 'boat train'. Do not worry if you are on the 'boat train' and you are delayed past the sailing time of the ferry. Depending upon the nature and length of the delay, the ferry will await the arrival of the 'boat train'. The reverse is also the case, as the advertised 'boat train' will await the arrival of the ferry.

FURTHER READING

- *Holidays and Travel Abroad 1990/91,* published by RADAR, price £2.00.

- *Holiday in the British Isles 1990,* publichsed by RADAR, price £3.00.

- *Access at the Channel Ports,* published by RADAR, price £2.75 inc. p & p.

TAXIS

Brian Howard

'Let's take a taxi' is a phrase few of us think of using when it comes to going out. Many people still think of taxis as a means of transport only for the businessman or the well-off.

But taxis are rapidly becoming an every-day part of public transport, along with buses, trains and planes. Some bus companies are already using taxibuses on routes where there is not enough demand for the usual larger buses, and some health authorities are now using taxis, instead of ambulances, to take people to and from hospital out-patient appointments.

This chapter looks at the useful part taxis can play in organising your journeys, the advantages they can bring, and the pitfalls to avoid. 'Taxis' and 'private-hire cars' (sometimes called 'minicabs') are both included here, and the difference between them explained, because they both give the same sort of service: your own door-to-door transport, available when you want it.

When to take a taxi

Compared with other transport, taxis and private-hire cars have a number of advantages:

They are generally available 24 hours a day, every day of the year (they are there when other public transport has stopped running).

You can usually hire one immediately you need one, or book one in advance (you are not bound by a timetable, as with buses and trains).

They provide a door-to-door service, so you can be picked up where you wish to be collected and taken to your exact destination (you don't have to walk to bus stops or find your own way from the station).

They are more convenient if you have heavy luggage or bulky parcels to take with you (you don't have to struggle on and off crowded buses and trains).

You can probably travel more comfortably than on buses or trains (you don't have crowds to cope with, or worry whether you will get a seat).

As an alternative to using your own car, you have no stress of driving, and no parking problems.

Of course you have to pay a price for the convenience of using taxis or private-hire cars. They are naturally more expensive than buses or trains, especially if you have a travel pass or tokens, which give you either free or cheap bus and rail journeys. Nevertheless, there are occasions when it makes economic sense to use a taxi or private-hire car (see Example 3 on page 36), and there are likely to be times when you would prefer the comfort and convenience of a taxi.

Because fares are based on the distance travelled, taxis are best used for short trips: to your nearest town, local hospital or shopping centre, or as part of a longer journey – to and from the station, or between stations if you need to get across London or other large cities.

You would not normally think of using taxis instead of long-distance coach or rail journeys.

Bearing this in mind, it would be worth considering using taxis or private-hire cars:

If there are two or more of you travelling (most taxis are licensed to carry up to five passengers and private-hire cars can usually take up to four). The cost is the same as, or only very slightly dearer than, for one person. Dividing the fare between you can make an otherwise expensive trip more affordable.

If you are making an occasional, special trip (eg going on holiday). The taxi fare to and from the station will be small compared with the cost of the whole journey, and if you have luggage, or the weather is bad, you may think the convenience is worth the extra cost.

If there is a low fare scheme in your area, such as 'Taxicard' or if you can use tokens or vouchers issued by your local council towards the cost of taxi fares.

If you have a disability which makes using buses and trains difficult or impossible for you, and there is no 'dial-a-ride' service available.

If you decide that it is worth it, the next thing to decide is whether to take a taxi or a private-hire car.

Taxi or private hire?

The main difference between a taxi service and a private-hire car (or 'minicab') service is a legal one. The law allows you to hire a taxi from a taxi-rank or in the street, or to book one in advance, by telephone.

A private-hire car cannot be hailed in the street, or at a taxi-rank; IT MUST be booked in advance from the car hire company, either in person or by telephone, whether the car is needed five minutes, five hours or five days ahead.

OUTSIDE LONDON

Taxis and their drivers are licensed by your local district council. You can hire taxis to take you anywhere, but a driver is only legally obliged to take you to a destination in the district council area where he is licensed.

Each council has regulations which cover every aspect of taxi operation, including:

- the fares charged (via a meter in the taxi)
- the type of vehicle which can be used as a taxi
- regular maintenance and inspection of the taxi
- insurance for the taxi and its passengers
- the driver's conduct

Some councils have introduced a geographical test which drivers have to pass before they can get a licence.

Outside London many councils are insisting that new licences will only be given to taxis which are wheelchair-accessible – in practice the new London standard black cab. Already they are appearing on the streets of Manchester, Newcastle-upon-Tyne, Reading, Exeter, Colchester and Bath. There are advantages and disadvantages to think about with both the London-style taxi and the saloon car.

IN LONDON

Taxis and their drivers are licensed by the Metropolitan Police. Regulations are similar to those for areas outside London, except that:

Vehicles have to be London's famous 'black cabs' (although they are now sometimes a different colour).

They can always be hired in the street if they are showing their yellow 'for hire' sign.

Taxis can be hired to take you anywhere you wish, but a driver is only legally obliged to take you to a destination in the Metropolitan Police District up to 6 miles (20 miles if you hire a taxi at Heathrow Airport).

In London, since February 1989, all new taxis have to be able to carry passengers who use wheelchairs, in their wheelchair, without them having to transfer into the back seat of the taxi. By the year 2000 every single one of London's 15,000 taxis will have to be wheelchair-accessible.

Already you can be sure that, at London's main-line railway stations and at Heathrow Airport, you will not have to wait very long in the taxi queue before a wheelchair-accessible taxi turns up. Some of them – called the 'Metro' – look squarer or 'chunkier' than the traditional London cab, but others – the 'Fairway' – do not look any different from the outside, so it is best to ask the driver if in doubt.

Private-hire cars

MINICABS

Private-hire cars do not have to be licensed, but outside London 85 per cent of district councils do licence them. In London private-hire cars are currently not licensed at all, but the law may soon be changed to give some control over them.

Whilst private-hire cars may be operated through reputable companies, may be safely maintained and driven, and their drivers may have adequate 'hire and reward' insurance, there can be no guarantee of this unless they are properly licensed.

Because private-hire cars and drivers do not have to meet the same stringent conditions as taxis and taxi-drivers, and because they have to be booked in advance, their fares are usually a little cheaper than taxi fares. In London, however, for short journeys they may be more expensive.

Private-hire cars, although often known as 'minicabs' are usually large 4-door saloon cars. They are often private family cars which double up as hire-cars when the driver is working for hire. The type of vehicle used can also be a very important issue when deciding whether to take a taxi or a private-hire car.

London-style taxi

PROS

Many are wheelchair-accessible, with a wider door opening, a ramp for wheelchair users and wheelchair restraint and safety-belt for passengers.

They can take up to four other passengers.

There is plenty of leg room.

CONS

There is a high step up into the taxi (but research is going on to see if this can be overcome), which means you have to bend your head and knee at the same time when you get in and out. You might worry about falling forwards into the taxi.

Larger electric wheelchairs may not be able to fit in the taxi and there may not be sufficient headroom if you are tall and have to sit upright in your wheelchair.

4-door saloon car

PROS

You may find it easier to get in and out if stepping up into a London-style taxi is too difficult for you.

CONS

You cannot travel in the vehicle in your wheelchair, if you use one (but larger saloon cars can take a folded-up wheelchair in the boot, if you can transfer to the car seat, using a transfer-board).

The seats are low down, which may make getting up out of the car difficult for you.

There is limited leg room.

With both types of vehicle taxi drivers are not obliged to help you from your door to the taxi or car, but most will help you into and out of the vehicle if you need assistance.

Taxi charges

Taxis and private-hire cars both charge according to distance. Taxis all have a meter (which cannot be tampered with) which shows the fare being charged. The amount shown goes up as the distance increases. Whilst you can get a rough idea from the driver beforehand what the fare will be, he must charge you the amount shown on the meter at the end of the trip.

There is usually a small extra charge for additional passengers (more than one), or for hiring at night-time, weekends and public holidays.

Private-hire car charges

Private-hire cars do not have meters (or, if they do, they do not have to be set at the taxi rate), and you should ask at the time of hiring what the charge will be. In fact, many advertise that they are metered at rates set by the local council.

Cost per mile

Because fare levels vary from town to town, and because fare increases for taxis are approved from time to time, it is impossible to give a fare-table here. However, as a very approximate guide only, you could assume it will cost around £1 per mile to hire a taxi, perhaps a bit less for a private-hire car (and remember you can travel with up to four others for virtually the same fare).

TIPPING

It is usual for the driver to expect a tip, of 10 per cent to 12.5 per cent of the fare, but do not feel pressured into giving a tip.

Help with taxi fares

OUTSIDE LONDON

Many councils offer cheap or free fare schemes for older users of public transport. Vouchers or tokens are supplied and sometimes these can also be used for taxi trips, using local taxi companies. Some areas, notably Edinburgh and the Central Region of Scotland, have introduced a Taxicard scheme specifically for disabled people, who cannot use buses or trains, or can only do so with great difficulty. These taxi trips are available to Taxicard holders at a much lower cost.

For further details of what, if any, concessionary fare schemes are available in your area, you should contact the department which deals with public transport matters at your county council offices (or regional council offices in Scotland).

Help with taxi fares

IN LONDON

The London Taxicard Scheme is open to disabled people who live in London (but not to visitors to London) who are seriously handicapped in their use of buses or trains. There is a minimum charge of £1.25 per trip but the scheme allows a saving, currently up to a maximum of £7.75 on each taxi journey.

This scheme is run for 30 of London's borough councils by London Transport's Unit for Disabled Passengers (see p 155). The taxis are provided by London's radio taxi companies so you can telephone for a taxi when you need one.

Further details and application forms for membership can be obtained from London Transport, council offices and post offices in the London boroughs unless you live in the City of Westminster, or in the boroughs of Redbridge or Barnet. These councils run their own Taxicard scheme and you need to apply to the social services department of the council, if you live in one of these areas.

Complaints

If you do have a complaint about the fare or about a taxi-driver you should:

> Raise the matter with the driver. If you are not satisfied with the result you should then:

> Complain to the taxi or private-hire company.

If you are still dissatisfied, or in the case of a serious complaint, you should then:

> Outside London – complain direct to the district council taxi licensing office,

> or

> In London – complain direct to the Public Carriage Office at: 15 Penton Street, London N1 9PU. Tel: 071-278 1744.

You will need to have as many details as possible:

1 The date and time of the booking;
2 The date and time of the journey;
3 The name of the taxi company;
4 Where the taxi picked you up and where it took you;
5 The taxi licence number, or the driver's licence no.

NB. If you have a complaint about an unlicensed private-hire car or minicab you will not be able to follow it up with the licensing authority, as these are outside their control.

TRAINS
Paul Salveson

Those who have not used the train for a while might be surprised about many of the improvements British Rail (BR) have made to its services, and at the cheap fare offers which are available. Most of this section is concerned with longer distance travel. Generally, you will find that BR's InterCity services are more comfortable than local and provincial services.

Railcards

If you are thinking about doing even one long(ish) rail journey, it will almost certainly pay you to get a 'Senior Railcard'. It costs just £16 for a year, and is available for both men and women aged 60 or over. For that, you get discounts of between a half and a third off the normal rail fares.

You can get a slightly better deal if you qualify for a Disabled Person's Railcard – ask BR for the leaflet which explains who is eligible. This card costs only £12 and gives you roughly the same discounts as the Senior Railcard.

Types of ticket

The most common ticket for longer journeys is the Saver – you get a third off the price, but try to avoid travelling on a Friday because it is more expensive.

If you live in the London area, and want to go to Newcastle to visit friends, it would cost £34.30 (return) each if you travelled any day except Friday (or Saturdays in July and August).

If you live in Greater Manchester, and wanted a day out in London, the cheapest fare with your railcard is £14.50. For shorter journeys, of less than 50 miles, you can get a cheap day return at half price with your railcard.

If you live in Manchester, and fancy a trip to Blackpool, it would cost you £2.85 each, and you even get some free tickets for the Pleasure Beach.

This is not a bad deal, and what is even better is that you can take your grandchildren along (or someone else's) at a set price of £1 each for up to four of them, on top of your own discount.

A leaflet on the Senior Railcard is available from most stations, and gives you further details and an application form. Take the completed form to a major BR station or rail-appointed travel agent, together with proof of your age (eg a passport, medical card, or birth certificate).

Leisurely trains

You do not have to use the train just to get from one place to another. Many find the train journey itself delightful, especially if it includes spectacular scenery (eg Settle – Carlisle line; West Highlands line from Glasgow to Fort William and Mallaig; Mid-Wales line from Shrewsbury to Swansea).

BR produce a range of leaflets on particular lines that appeal to the leisure traveller. The Rail Rover tickets (with extra discounts for railcard holders) are especially good value: the 'Freedom of the Coast and Peaks' ticket, covering an area from North Wales to Shropshire, the Peak District and Manchester, costs £20 for unlimited travel for seven days (with a railcard: £13.20).

Concessionary fares

Check whether you can make local train journeys using your concessionary fare pass. Where this facility is available, it is often cheaper than travelling on a railcard ticket.

Group travel

There are fare reductions for group travel. If there are a lot of you, you can even charter your own train.

Planning your journey

When you take your railcard application form down to the station or travel agent, it should be possible for you to book your rail tickets at the same time. When you are intending to go on a longer journey or have an appointment at the other end, try to buy your tickets in advance. Although it is perfectly easy to buy tickets on the day, a long queue may make you miss your train and you will certainly be too late to reserve a seat.

WHICH DAY WILL YOU TRAVEL?

Monday to Thursday are the best days to travel. If you can, avoid Friday and Saturday, as both are busy and Friday is more expensive. Sunday timetables are sometimes disrupted, due to engineering work on the tracks, which could make your journey a bit frustrating. This is not to say that weekends are to be avoided, just that you should check if there have been any alterations to the published train services.

WHAT TIME DO YOU WANT TO ARRIVE?

The BR staff will advise you which is the best service to get, and the connections if you have to change trains. First of all, you need to decide when you want to arrive, especially if someone is meeting you at the other end.

DO YOU NEED TO BOOK A SEAT?

Ask BR staff if it is advisable to reserve a seat. On longer journeys, it is worth doing this as a matter of course. It only costs £1 to reserve seats for up to four people travelling together. Seat reservations are now compulsory on certain services at particularly busy times of the year.

WILL THERE BE CATERING FACILITIES?

Virtually all InterCity trains now have catering facilities of some kind, as do longer distance provincial services. However, they usually charge more than average cafe prices, so if you are on a tight budget bring your own sandwiches.

Boarding

It is always best to double-check with platform staff that you have the right train. If the station is not staffed, ask the conductor on the train when it pulls in (he or she will usually be at the rear end of the train).

Alighting

If you are leaving the train before its final destination, it is a good idea to find out the name of the previous stop to your own, so you can be ready in good time. Very often, the conductor will announce the station as the train approaches. It does no harm to ask the conductor to let you know when you are near your stop. Never leave the train or open the door until the train has come to a complete halt, and if necessary ask platform staff for assistance.

If things go wrong

If your train is running so late that you are going to miss your connection, speak to the conductor and it may be possible to hold the connecting train until your train arrives. If you are unlucky enough to miss your last train home, due to your own train being delayed, BR will get you home somehow – or put you up overnight.

Frailty and disability

Bearing in mind that much of the rail network was built in the last century, it is hardly surprising stations often have poor accessibility – steps, footbridges, steep ramps and the like – for people with mobility difficulties.

If you have mobility difficulties, make this clear to the staff, in advance, when you are booking your ticket and during the journey. Make sure that enough time has been left for connections to be made during the trip. If you need assistance with a wheelchair, BR will arrange the necessary help at departure and arrival, but insist that they are informed in advance.

BR are gradually improving the situation. Whilst most trains – and all InterCity services – have toilet facilities, toilets accessible to wheelchair users are still being introduced, as and when new rolling stock is purchased or old stock refurbished. Only a few local trains are still without toilets. Spaces near to accessible toilets are available on InterCity and provincial trains.

At stations, BR are installing induction loops in all its booking offices, so that you can use a hearing aid with a 'T' switch. Goods lifts can sometimes be used to help you get from platform to platform, but BR require a member of staff to be present to operate them. BR have a portable ramp which can be attached to train doorways, designed mainly with wheelchair users in mind.

Complaints

If there is something wrong with the train itself – toilet out of order, offensive passengers – speak in the first instance with the conductor. If anything happens which you consider to be BR's fault, complain about it to your BR Area Manager. If you get no satisfaction, you can seek redress through the Transport Users' Consultative Committee. Both the Manager and the Committee's addresses are displayed on wall posters at BR stations.

CASE HISTORY

Chris and Julie Traynor live in Penzance, Cornwall and go to visit their friend in London. They decide to go by train (return fare, with Railcard, £31.70 each) and the journey takes five hours. Going by car would have taken too long (about seven hours, with stops for meals and a rest), and they would have had to drive through London at the end. The coach would have been cheaper (return fare, £17 each) but would have taken seven hours forty minutes, so they prefer to go for speed and comfort.

They telephone the station to find out the train times and ask whether they need to book seats. They are told that there will be plenty of room on their particular service. Chris packs a few sandwiches and a flask, although there is a buffet service on board. They get a taxi to the station because it is more convenient than taking a bus or their car (and

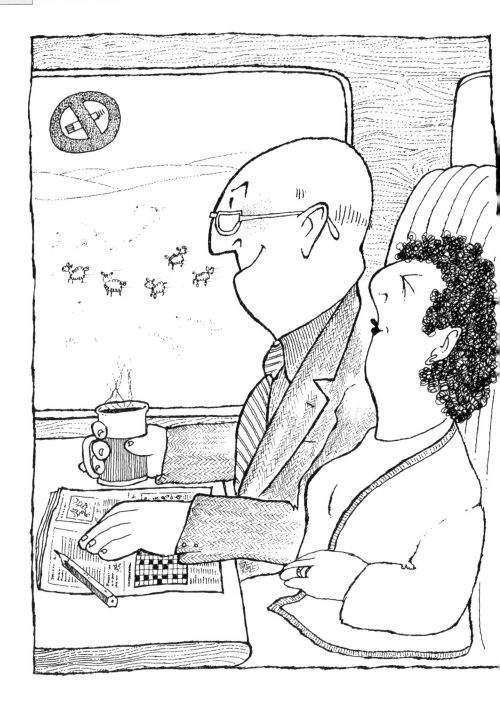

they would worry if it stood in a car park for a week). They time their journey to arrive in London before the evening rush hour (3.30 pm) and – still using the ticket they bought at home – they catch the Underground across London to their friend's house.

In both instances the common factor is the need to plan: any journey needs to be worked out, with all the right information. The simplest way to get this information is to go down to a BR travel centre. If you cannot do that, look BR up in the phone book and ring 'Passenger Information'.

WALKING

Barbara Preston

Walking is the most basic method of getting about. It is particularly important for four reasons:

1 It promotes physical health
Recent research has shown that people who are active are healthier and less likely to die of heart disease and a range of other illnesses than those who take less exercise. Walking is a good way of keeping active.

2 It prevents isolation
Walking is the chief method of keeping in touch with neighbours, either through visiting or the informal chat when out shopping.

3 It gives independence
If you can still walk to the shops, to the library, to the doctor and for other essential services, you retain your independence.

4 It's free
After the initial outlay on footwear and waterproof clothing, walking is the cheapest way to travel.

It is important, therefore, to keep walking even if it is not as easy as it was. Perhaps more important, because it is less obvious, if you still drive a car everywhere, think about making some trips on foot, so that you develop the walking habit and stay independent.

Plan your route

Plan your route before you start and never attempt to cross the road where you cannot see whether the road is clear in both directions. Do not cross at bends where the sight lines are bad for both pedestrian and driver. Plan ahead so that you do not have to cross at a dangerous place.

Pedestrian crossings

If there is any particular danger spot in your area try to get it improved by contacting your local authority or your local councillor. For instance, you may feel that the road is so busy that there is a need for a pedestrian crossing facility, a zebra or a pelican crossing or a 'green man' phase at the traffic lights.

The criterion for a pelican or zebra crossing is based on the number of people crossing a road per hour against the number of vehicles driving on that road per hour. The total is averaged over the busiest four-hour period. The number of people multiplied by the square of the number of vehicles should be equal to or over one hundred million.

If the traffic flow is 600 vehicles per hour then 300 people per hour must cross the road to satisfy this criterion; if there are 1,000 vehicles per hour a crossing would be justified for 100 people crossing the road. If there are special circumstances, such as an old people's home, or sheltered accommodation in the vicinity, then crossing facilities might be provided even if this figure is not reached.

Whether the authorities will provide pedestrian facilities at traffic signalled junctions will depend partly on whether they are likely to cause traffic congestion and partly on how many people have been injured at that junction.

You may well feel that you have not got sufficient time to cross the road at a pelican crossing. New regulations introduced in 1987 enable a local authority to increase the 'steady green man' period of time up to nine seconds on wide roads. If you can persuade the local authority that this is necessary there is no reason why this longer time should not be introduced.

Look after yourself

Everyone has the right to walk, which includes crossing the road, but it is no use your trying to prove your right by pitting yourself against a vehicle.

It is particularly dangerous to cross the road near to, but not at, a pelican crossing. You should cross on the crossing but you should still take care; over half of those injured on pelican crossings were crossing correctly, starting to cross during the 'steady green man' period. So, even if you cross then, watch out for traffic, as the driver may not stop.

When you go out after dark make sure that drivers can see you. You may well be able to see them, but can they see you? In Scandinavian countries, where pedestrian casualty rates are much lower than in Britain, people out in the dark customarily wear reflecting discs. Reflecting stickers can be bought from Nord Associates Limited (see p 156), and put onto handbags, walking sticks, shoes, clothing and the dog's collar. The Royal Society for the Prevention of Accidents (RoSPA) (see p 156) and some local authorities also sell reflecting stickers (ask for the Road Safety Section). But remember that even if the driver has seen you it is up to you to keep out of the way; the driver may well assume that you are going to get out of the way and so may not slow down, or may not be able to stop in time.

Walking for pleasure

There are now a range of organisations, commercial and otherwise such as Campus Travel (see p 156), arranging walking holidays, both in Britain and abroad. The Ramblers' Association (see p 156) organises local walks and seeks to protect walkers' access to the countryside. Outdoor pursuits shops will often have contact with local rambling clubs or groups.

Frailty and disability

As outlined in the earlier section on Mobility Aids (see p 113), there are many ways of keeping on the move, even when you are less agile than you were.

After a hip operation one leg may be shorter than the other. Raised shoes are needed and once you know the extra height necessary a shoe repairer can add the extra height to the required heel, even on your best shoes. Surgical shoes are supplied by hospitals, free under the National Health Service but only one pair a year is allowed.

People who have problems with their feet should consult a chiropodist. Chiropody treatment is free under the National Health Service for pensioners. All chiropodists working for health authorities must be State Registered. If you go privately make sure that the chiropodist you visit is State Registered, with the letters S.R.Ch. after the name.

Complaints

For people who are visually impaired it is important that there are no unexpected obstructions on the pavement. Cars parked on the pavement can be particularly hazardous. Nationally it is not an offence to park on the pavement, though in some places, notably in London, local authorities have introduced by-laws to make this an offence. Thanks to the wording of the 1835 Highway Act, it is an offence punishable by a fine of up to £10 – quite a lot in those days – to wilfully lead or drive any horse, ass, sheep, mule, swine or cattle, or carriage of any description on any footpath by the side of the road. Since a car parked on the footway will, almost always, have been driven there it is possible to prosecute under the 1835 Act and this has been done successfully in some areas.

There is also the problem that motor vehicles, particularly heavy vehicles, may cause considerable damage to the surface of the pavement and broken and uneven paving stones can be dangerous. Street furniture, piles of dust bin bags, cycles and motorcycles fastened to the inside of guard rails and goods displayed outside shops can also be dangerous. Poor lighting can also make journeys at night a problem.

If you suffer inconvenience from any of these things, and especially if you have suffered any injury from them, get in touch with your local authority. However, if your local authority is unhelpful or unsympathetic, contact the Pedestrians' Association (see p 156).

PART 3

Further information *This section provides a useful list of organisations and companies mentioned in Parts 1 and 2. While Out and About sets out to give a general view about travel these contacts will help you with specific enquiries when planning your journey.*

Useful addresses

PLANNING

Youth Hostels Assocation
(Membership, Youth Hostel
Information)
Trevelyan House
8 St Stephens Hill
St Albans AL1 2DY
Tel: 0727 40211

ACCESS

AA (Automobile Association)
Fanum House
Basingstoke
Hampshire RG21 2EA
Tel: 0256 20123

AA Publications Centre
Distribution Service
Dunhams Lane
Letchworth
Hertfordshire SG6 1LF
Tel: 0462 686241

The English Tourist Board
Thames Tower
Blacks Road
London W6 9EL
Tel: 081-846 9000

Holiday Care Service
2 Old Bank Chambers
Station Road
Horley
Surrey RH6 9HW
Tel: 0293 774535

Museums and Galleries Commission
7 St. James's Square
London SW1Y 4JU
Tel: 071-839 9341

National Gardens Scheme
Hatchlands Park
East Clandon
Guildford
Surrey GU4 7RT
Tel: 0483 211535

National Trust
36 Queen Anne's Gate
London SW1H 9AS
Tel: 071-222 9251

National Trust for Scotland
5 Charlotte Square
Edinburgh EH2 4DU
Tel: 031-226 5922

RADAR
(The Royal Association for
Disability and Rehabilitation)
25 Mortimer Street
London W1N 8AB
Tel: 071-637 5400

RSPB
(The Royal Society for the
Protection of Birds)
The Lodge, Sandy
Bedfordshire SG19 2DL
Tel: 0767 680551

MONEY

Association of British Travel Agents (ABTA)
55-57 Newman Street,
London W1P 4AH
Tel: 071-637 2444

AIR TRAVEL

British Airports Authority
130 Wilton Road
London SW1V 1LQ
Tel: 071-834 9449

British Airways
P.O. Box 10
Heathrow Airport
Hounslow,
Middlesex TW6 2JA
Tel: 081-897 4000

Flightlink
294 Soho Road
Birmingham B21 9LY
Tel: 021-554 5232

Gatwick Travel Care
Room 3058
Gatwick Airport
South Terminal
Gatwick
West Sussex RH6 0NP
Tel: 0293 28822 x 4283

Heathrow Travel Care
Room 1214
Queens Building (1st Floor)
Heathrow Airport
Hounslow
Middlesex TW6 1JH
Tel: 081-745 7495

BUSES

Bus and Coach Council
Sardinia House
52 Lincoln's Inn Fields
London WC2A 3LZ
Tel: 071-831 7546

**Buswatch
(Bus Passengers' Monitoring Project)**
18 Little Southsea Street
Southsea
Hampshire PO5 3RS
Tel: 0705 863080

National Federation of Bus Users
The Secretary
6 Holmhurst Lane
St. Leonards-on-Sea
East Sussex TN37 7LW
Tel: 0424 752424

CARS

A.I.D. Vehicle Supplies
Hockley Industrial Estate Centre
Hooley Lane
P.O. Box 26
Redhill
Surrey RH1 6JF
Tel: 0737 770030

**BVRLA
(British Vehicle Rental and Leasing Association)**
13 St John's Street
Chichester
West Sussex PO19 1UU
Tel: 0243 786782

DSS
Disablement Services Branch
Block 1
Government Buildings
Warbreck Hill Road
Blackpool FY2 0UZ

DVLC
(Driver and Vehicle Licensing Centre)
Swansea SA99 1BN
Tel: 0792 72151

Mobility Advice and Vehicle Information Service (MAVIS)
TRRL
Crowthorne
Berkshire RG11 6AU
Tel: 0344 770456

Motability
Gate House
2nd Floor
West Gate
Harlow
Essex CM20 1HR
Tel: 0279 635666

Royal Automobile Club
Marco Polo House
3-5 Lansdowne Road
Croydon CR9 2JH
Tel: 081-686 2314

Continental Motorail Services
Contact:
The Car Ferry Centre
Terminal House
21-23 Elizabeth Street
London SW1W RRP
Tel: 071-730 3440

Insurance organisations specialising in policies for older drivers

Age Concern Insurance Services
Garrod House
Chaldon Road
Caterham CR3 5YZ
Tel: 0883 346964

Refuge Assurance plc
Refuge House
Alderley Road
Wilmslow
Cheshire SK9 1PF
Tel: 0625 535959

Insurance organisations specialising in policies for disabled drivers

Gibb Hartley Cooper Limited
Chartis Tower
Dock Street
Newport
Gwent NP9 1DW
Tel: 0633 250222

M J Fish and Co
1-3 Slater Lane
Leyland
Preston
Lancashire PR5 3AL
Tel: 0772 455111

Chartwell Insurance Brokers
Incorporating:
Disabled Drivers Insurance Bureau
292 Hale Lane
Edgeware
Middlesex HA8 8NP
Tel: 081-958 3135

L Hughes and Co
48 Frances Street
Newtownards
County Down
Northern Ireland BT23 3DN
Tel: 0247 817375

Consumer Insurance Services
2 Osborns Court
High Street South
Olney
Buckinghamshire MK46 4AA
Tel: 0234 713535

Amicable Insurance Consultants
39 The High Street
Crawley
West Sussex RH10 1BK
Tel: 0293 561233

COACHES

Armstrong Galley
120 Northumberland Street
Newcastle upon Tyne NE1 7DG
Tel: 091-232 3918

Bus and Coach Council
Sardinia House
52 Lincoln's Inn Fields
London WC2A 3LZ
Tel: 071-381 7546

Caledonian Express
Walnut Grove
Perth PH2 7LP
Tel: 0738 33481

National Express
4 Vicarage Road
Edgbaston

Birmingham B15 3ES
Tel: 021-456 1122
(London 071-730 0202)
Also check the phone book,
Yellow Pages and Thomsons
Directory for local enquiry
numbers; there are about 3,000
offices and agents.

Scottish Citylink Coaches Ltd
Buchanan Bus Station
Killermont Street
Glasgow G2 3NP
Tel: 041-332 9644
(London office 071-636 9373)

West Midlands Travel
Central-Liner
Newton Coach Terminal
Miller Street
Birmingham B6 4NG
Tel: 021-236 8313

COMMUNITY TRANSPORT

British Red Cross Society
9 Grosvenor Crescent
London SW1X 7EJ
Tel: 071-235 5454

Community Transport Association
Highbank
Halton Street
Hyde
Cheshire SK14 2NY
Tel: 061-351 1475

London Community Transport Association
Interchange Studios
15 Wilkin Street
London NW5 3NG
Tel: 071-284 4600

Tripscope
63 Esmond Road
London W4 IJE
Tel: 081-994 9294

Women's Royal Voluntary Service (WRVS)
234/244 Stockwell Road
London SW9 9SP
Tel: 071-416 0146

CYCLING

Cyclists' Touring Club
Cotterell House
69 Meadrow
Godalming
Surrey GU7 3HS
Tel: 04868 7217

Fellowship of Cycling Old Timers
c/o Jim Shaw
2 Westwood Road
Marlow
Buckinghamshire SL7 2AT

A loose association of people with long cycling memories, which produces a quarterly newsletter for its members.

NOTE: The **Veterans' Cycling Club**, is a club for people with veteran cycles, NOT veteran cyclists, although they do have

15 to 20 members over 70 and half a dozen over 80.

London Cycling Campaign
3 Stamford Street
London SE1 9NT
Tel: 071-928 7220

Susi Madron's Cycling for Softies
Lloyds House
22 Lloyd Street
Manchester M2 5WA
Tel: 061-834 6800

GOING ABROAD

Consular Department
Foreign and Commonwealth Office
Clive House
Petty France
London SW1H 9HD
Tel: 071-270 3000

Medical Advisory Service for Travellers Abroad (MASTA)
London School of Hygiene and Tropical Medicine
Keppel Street
London WC1E 7HT
Tel: 071-631 4408

LONDON

London City Airport
King George V Dock
Silvertown
London E16 2PX
Tel: 071-474 5555

**London Regional
Passengers' Committee**
Golden Cross House
8 Duncannon Street
London WC2N 4JF
Tel: 071-839 1898

London Transport
Travel Information Service
55 Broadway
London SW1H OBD
Tel: 071-222 1234

Riverbus
Exchange Tower
1 Harbour Exchange Square
London E14 9GE
Tel: 071-512 0555

Unit for Disabled Passengers
The Unit's phone number is
071-222 5600 or you can write to:

Unit for Disabled Passengers
London Transport
55 Broadway
London SW1H 0BD

MOBILITY AIDS
Banstead Place Mobility Centre
Park Road
Banstead
Surrey SM7 3EE
Tel: 0737 351674

**HM Customs and Excise
Department**
New Kings Beam House
22 Upper Ground
London SE1 9PJ
Tel: 071-620 1313

**National Federation of
Shopmobility**
17 Grange Place
Grange Town
Cardiff CF1 7DB
Tel: 0222 236255

Disabled Living Foundation
380-384 Harrow Road
London W9 2HU
Tel: 071-289 6111

**RADAR
(Royal Association
for Disability and
Rehabilitation)**
25 Mortimer Street
London W1N 8AB
Tel: 071-637 5400

SEA TRAVEL
B&I Line (UK) Limited
Passenger Office
Reliance House
Water Street
Liverpool L28 2TP
Tel: 051-227 3131

Caledonian Macbrayne Limited
The Ferry Terminal
Gourock PA19 1QP
Tel: 0475 34531

British Ports Association
Victoria House
Vernon Place
London WC1
Tel: 071-242 1200

Disabled Drivers' Assocation
Drake House
18 Creekside
London SE8 3DZ
Tel: 081-692 7141

Disabled Drivers' Motoring Club
Cottingham Way
Thrapston
Northamptonshire NN14 4PL
Tel: 0801 24724

Scandinavian Seaways
Scandinavia House
Parkeston Quay
Harwich
Essex CO12 4QG
Tel: 0255 240240
Reservations (Auto queuing)
0255 243456
Port Office:
also DFDS Travel Centre
15 Hanover Street
London W1R 9HG
Tel: 071-493 6696

Sealink
16 Monmouth Street
London WC2H 9HB
Tel: 071-836 9421

Nord Associates Limited
St. Peters School House
Sparty Lea
Near Hexham
Northumberland NE47 9UN
Tel: 0434 685351

The Pedestrians Association
1 Wandsworth Road
London SW8 2XX
Tel: 071-735 3270

Ramblers' Association
1-5 Wandsworth Road
London SW8 2XX
Tel: 071-582 6878

Royal Society for the Prevention of Accidents (RoSPA)
Road Safety Division
Cannon House
The Priory
Queensway
Birmingham B4 6BS
Tel: 021-200 2461

WALKING

Campus Travel
166 Deansgate
Manchester M3 3FE
Tel: 061-833 2046

Organise walking holidays, in conjunction with the Youth Hostel Association, for people of all ages.

About Age Concern

Out and About is one of a wide range of titles published by Age Concern England – the National Council on Ageing. In addition, Age Concern England is actively engaged in training, information provision, research and campaigning for retired people and those who work with them. It is a registered charity dependent on public support for the continuation of its work. Age Concern England links closely with Age Concern centres in Scotland, Wales and Northern Ireland to form a network of over 1,400 independent local UK groups. These groups, with the invaluable help of an estimated 250,000 volunteers, aim to improve the quality of life for older people and develop services appropriate to local needs and resources. These include advice and information, day care, visiting services, transport schemes, clubs and specialist facilities for physically and mentally frail older people.

Age Concern England
1268 London Road
London SW16 4ER
Tel: 081-679 8000

Age Concern Scotland
54A Fountainbridge
Edinburgh EH3 9PT
Tel: 031-228 5656

Age Concern Wales
4th Floor
1 Cathedral Road
Cardiff CF1 9SD
Tel: 0222 371821/371566

Age Concern Northern Ireland
6 Lower Crescent
Belfast BT7 1NR
Tel: 0232 245729

Publications from Age Concern

A wide range of titles is published under the Age Concern imprint.

MONEY MATTERS

Using Your Home as Capital
Cecil Hinton

This best-selling book for home-owners, which is updated annually, gives a detailed explanation of how to capitalise on the value of your home and obtain a regular additional income.

0-86242-096-2   Price on application

Your Taxes and Savings
John Burke, Joanna Hanks and Simon Richmond

The complexities of our tax system as they affect older people are explained in straightforward terms in this invaluable annual guide.

0-86242-093-8   Price on application

Your Rights
Sally West

A highly acclaimed annual guide to the State benefits available to older people. Contains current information on Income Support, Housing Benefit and Retirement Pensions among other matters and provides advice on how to claim them.

0-86242-089-X   Price on application

Managing Other People's Money
Penny Letts

The management of money and property is usually a personal and private matter. However, there may come a time when someone else has to take over on either a temporary or permanent basis. This book looks at the circumstances in which such a need could arise and provides a step-by-step guide to the arrangements which have to be made.

£5.95   0-86242-090-3

GENERAL

Living, Loving and Ageing: Sexual and personal relationships in later life

Wendy Greengross and Sally Greengross

Sexuality is often regarded as the preserve of the younger generation. At last, here is a book for older people, and those who work with them, which tackles the issues in a straightforward fashion, avoiding preconceptions and bias.

£4.95   0-86242-070-9

Famous Ways to Grow Old

Philip Bristow

A collection of letters from a host of internationally distinguished figures, outlining their personal attitudes to the onset of old age. Full of amusing and touching anecdotal material. Contributors include: James Callaghan; Peggy Ashcroft; Cardinal Basil Hume and Barbara Cartland.

£8.95   0-86242-087-3

Life in the Sun: A guide to long-stay holidays and living abroad in retirement

Nancy Tuft

Every year millions of older people consider either taking long-stay holidays or moving abroad on a more permanent basis. This essential guide examines the pitfalls associated with such a move and tackles topics varying from pets to Poll Tax.

£6.95   0-86242-085-7

HOUSING

A Buyer's Guide to Sheltered Housing
Age Concern England and the NHTPC

Buying a flat or bungalow in a sheltered scheme? This guide provides vital information on the running costs, design and management of schemes to help you make an informed decision.
£2.50   0-86242-063-6

At Home in a Home
Pat Young

The questions older people ask when considering moving into residential accommodation are answered in this practical guide. Such topics as fees, financial support and standards of care are tackled in realistic terms in order to help people make the right choice.
£3.95   0-86242-062-8

Housing Options for Older People
David Bookbinder

A review of housing options is part of growing older. All the possibilities and their practical implications are carefully considered in this comprehensive guide.
£2.50   0-86242-055-5

An Owner's Guide: Your Home in Retirement
Age Concern England and the NHTPC

A guide to ways in which older owner-occupiers can make their homes more comfortable and easier to manage. Advice is given on topics such as repairs and maintenance, heating, insulation and home security. There is also information on adapting a home for disabled residents and the sort of grants available for such work.
£2.50   0-86242-095-4

HEALTH

Your Health in Retirement

Dr J A Muir Gray and Pat Blair

This book is a comprehensive source of information to help readers look after themselves and work towards better health. Produced in an accessible A-Z style, full details are given of people and useful organisations from which assistance can be sought.

£4.50   0-86242-082-2

Know Your Medicines

Pat Blair

This guide for older people and their carers explains how the body works and how it is affected by medication. Also included is guidance on using medicines and an index of commonly used medicines and their side effects.

£3.95   0-86242-043-1

The Foot Care Book: An A-Z of fitter feet

Judith Kemp SRCh

A self-help guide for older people on routine foot care, this book includes an A-Z of problems, information on adapting and choosing shoes and a guide to who's who in foot care.

£2.95   0-86242-066-0

In Control: Help with Incontinence

Penny Mares

Containing information about the nature and causes of incontinence and the sources of help available, this book has been written for anyone concerned about this problem, either professionally or at home. The text is illustrated throughout with diagrams and case histories.

£4.50   0-86242-088-1

PROFESSIONAL

Age: The Unrecognised Discrimination
Edited by Evelyn McEwen

Comprising a series of discussive essays by leading specialists on evidence of age discrimination in British society today, including the fields of employment, healthcare, leisure and the voluntary sector, this book is an important contribution to the growing debate.
£9.95   0-86242-094-6

A Warden's Guide to Healthcare in Sheltered Housing
Dr Anne Roberts

An invaluable guide for all wardens and care home proprietors on the health needs of older people and the best means of promoting better health for their residents.
£6.50   0-86242-052-0

Cooking for Elderly People
Alan Stewart

Designed for use by anyone catering for groups of older people. This excellent manual contains over 120 thoroughly tested recipes.
£17.50   0-86388-046-0

The Law and Vulnerable Elderly People
Edited by Sally Greengross

This report raises fundamental questions about the way society views and treats older people. The proposals put forward seek to enhance the self-determination and autonomy of vulnerable old people and to ensure that they are better protected in the future.
£6.50   0-06242-050-4

Old Age Abuse
Mervyn Eastman

This book looks at three main aspects of old age abuse; the setting, the victims and the solutions. The studies are based on the author's 14 years as a social work practitioner. He presents the frustrating

dilemma facing those people who act in violence to those whom they may love and the tragic consequences of these actions.
£5.00   0-86242-030-X

Taking Good Care: A handbook for care assistants
Jenyth Worsley

As the first book written specifically for care staff, this publication will quickly become the primary reference source for both public and private sectors. Produced in 'handbook' style, it deliberately avoids jargon and technical terms and presents the information in a highly accessible format, illustrated with many case histories. Topics covered include the role of the assistant, the resident's viewpoint, activities and groupwork, and the latest research into the ageing process.
£6.95   0-86242-072-5

If you would like to order any of these titles, please write to the address below, enclosing a cheque or money order for the appropriate amount. Credit card orders may be made on 081-679 8000.

Age Concern England (DEPT OAA)
1268 London Road
London SW16 4ER

Information Factsheets

Age Concern England produces factsheets on a variety of subjects. Among the 30 factsheets produced, the following titles may be of use to readers of this book:

Holidays for Older People   Factsheet No. 4

Raising Income or Capital from Your Home   Factsheet No. 12

Income Tax and Older People   Factsheet No. 15

Income Related Benefits: Income and Capital   Factsheet No. 16

Help with Incontinence   Factsheet No. 23

Travel Information for Older People   Factsheet No. 26

To order the factsheets:
Single copies are free on receipt of a 9" × 6" sae.

If you require a selection of factsheets or multiple copies, charges will be given on request.

A complete set of factsheets is available in a ring binder at the current cost of £24, which includes the first year's subscription. The current cost for an annual subscription for subsequent years is £10. There are different rates of subscription for people living abroad.

Factsheets are revised and updated throughout the year and membership of the subscription service will ensure that your information is always current.

Write to:
Information and Policy Department
Age Concern England
Astral House
1268 London Road
London SW16 4ER

We hope you found this book useful. If so, perhaps you would like to receive further information about Age Concern or help us do more for elderly people.

Dear Age Concern
Please send me the details I've ticked below:

other publications ☐   *Age Concern special offers* ☐

volunteer with a local group ☐   *regular giving* ☐

covenant ☐   *legacy* ☐

Meantime, here is a gift of

£ _____ PO/CHEQUE or VISA/ACCESS No _____

NAME (BLOCK CAPITALS) _____

SIGNATURE _____

ADDRESS _____

_____

_____ POSTCODE _____

Please pull out this page and send it to: **Age Concern** (DEPT OAA)
FREEPOST
1268 London Road
no stamp needed **London SW16 4BR**

About the Community Transport Association

The Community Transport Association is the representative body of community, voluntary and non-profit passenger transport operators in Britain, especially those running minibuses.

The travel and transport needs of over 10 per cent of the population are currently not being catered for by conventional means of transport. The Association seeks to promote good practice amongst all those who are trying to reduce these mobility difficulties.

The Association's main activities, which are mostly self-financing, are:

- Publishing, including *Community Transport Magazine, Your Minibus: Is It Legal?*, and the Driver Assessment and Training Pack
- Training Courses
- Conferences, including the Annual Community Transport Event
- Exhibitions, including the Annual Community Transport Show
- Services for members, including the CTA Vehicle Purchase Scheme, Minibus Permits, and Reversing Safety Equipment bought in bulk
- Advice and information.

The Association seeks to present its views on a wide range of legal, technical and financial matters to local and central government, the commercial companies supplying non-profit minibus operators, and other national voluntary organisations. With over 70,000 minibuses on the road, there is plenty to do!

Membership is open to individuals, community and voluntary transport groups, Age Concerns, local authorities, health authorities and other statutory bodies.

For a sample information pack, send a large (A4), self-addressed envelope, with two second class stamps to: The Secretary, Community Transport Association, Highbank, Halton Street, Hyde, Cheshire, SK14 2NY. Telephone: 061-351 1475.

About National Express

GET TOGETHER WITH NATIONAL EXPRESS

Coach travel, with its low fares and frequent services, is such great value for money. As the UK's largest operator of scheduled express coach services, National Express is in the ideal position of being able to offer you an unrivalled choice of around 1500 destinations from which to choose.

But who are National Express and just what do they have to offer?

The National Express coach network covers England, Scotland and Wales with services stretching from Cornwall up to the Scottish Highlands and from North Wales to Kent.

Most services run every day of the week, including Sundays, with timetables offering hourly departures on many routes. The National Express network runs every day of the year except Christmas Day (there's even a limited service on Boxing Day) with many routes offering overnight services giving early morning arrivals at your destination.

In Scotland, the National Express name changes to Caledonian Express but continues to offer the same high level of service. Caledonian Express coaches link most Scottish towns and cities and offer a direct link between Scotland and London using the very latest luxury double-deck coaches. Many Scottish destinations are served by direct coaches from other parts of England and Wales.

Travelling around the country couldn't be easier with National Express. If there isn't a direct coach going to your destination a simple change of coach at one of our main interchange points such as Birmingham, Bristol, Leeds, Manchester, Glasgow or Perth will ensure that you complete your journey with the minimum of fuss.

TAKING THE 'RAPIDE'

Most of the longer routes are now operated by our luxury 'Rapide' coaches offering the very latest in comfort and service. Each 'Rapide' coach carries a hostess or steward who will be able to serve a range of light refreshments to you in your seat and will be on-hand should you need any advice or assistance during your journey. 'Rapide' coaches are fitted with reclining seats, a toilet/washroom, curtains and individual air-conditioning.

With more and more people flying abroad for a break in the sun, the main National Express Airport services are becoming increasingly popular. There are direct services from most parts of the country to Heathrow, Gatwick, Luton and Manchester Airports. Other routes serve Birmingham, East Midlands and Bristol Airports. Most airport services are operated by 'Rapide' coaches giving you the chance to start your holiday even before you reach the airport.

HELPING THE OLDER TRAVELLER

In an average year, National Express and Caledonian Express carry around 14 million passengers, a high proportion of these being over 50. For the older traveller with more time to spare, taking the coach becomes a very attractive way of travelling around the country and National Express is able to offer special assistance to anyone who may feel unsure about their travel arrangements.

Booking a ticket is simplicity itself. There are around 2,500 National Express appointed agents in England and Wales and around 450 in Scotland. These agents include main booking offices in bus and coach stations, high street travel agents and small village shops. Each agent holds full details of all National Express and Caledonian Express services and is able to issue a ticket to any destination on the coach network.

If you are travelling alone or have a disability and would like assistance when either joining or leaving your coach, this can be arranged at the same time as you book your ticket. It is, however, important to note that seven days notice is usually required and assistance may only be available at the larger bus and coach stations.

National Express and Caledonian Express fares offer exceptional value for money when compared with other forms of travel. Anyone aged 60 or over is entitled to a discount of around 30 per cent off the normal fare. Fares are usually higher for journeys made on a Friday (and also on Saturdays in July and August). Return tickets are valid for up to three months. A Reserved ticket can be bought in advance for any journey although if you decided to travel at the last minute, a Stand-by ticket is available at a reduced price.

Telephone bookings can be made using Access and Visa although five clear days notice is required to allow time for the ticket to be posted on to you.

THE NEW 'EXPRESSLINER' COACH

Today's modern coaches are a far cry from the old charabancs of yesteryear. A new type of single-deck coach, known as the 'Expressliner', is currently entering service on National Express and Caledonian Express routes throughout the UK. The 'Expressliner' carries several new features that are already making it easier for everyone using the coach.

The 'Expressliner' is fitted with a 'kneeling' suspension which automatically lowers the front of the coach once it has come to a stop. This lower front step and brightly coloured grab rails now make it much easier to get on and off the coach. Inside, a new design of toilet/washroom, a new servery for use by the hostess or steward, reclining seats, individual air conditioning, curtains, moveable footrests, airline style overhead luggage lockers and seat-back trays mean that you will complete your journey in absolute comfort. The 'Expressliner' also carries the very latest safety systems including a new braking system and a speed limiter, all designed to ensure that you reach your destination safely and in comfort.

TAKING THE FAMILY PET

Taking the family pet along with you on your journey can sometimes be a headache. Small dogs or other small domestic animals will normally be carried on National Express and Caledonian Express services provided they are accompanied. However, for reasons of hygiene, no animals will be carried on 'Rapide' services or any other service, indicated in the public timetable, where refreshments are served. It is also advisable, again in the interests of comfort and hygiene, not to take any animal on a journey where there is a journey time of more than three hours between stops.

COACH AND BUS STATIONS

Facilities at bus and coach stations vary enormously around the country. Most of these are not owned by National Express and it is therefore the responsibility of the owner to keep the facilities in full working order. However, most bus and coach stations have been or are being modernised and offer a high level of customer facilities including toilets for the disabled, waiting rooms, telephones and refreshments. In most of the larger bus and coach stations a National Express or Caledonian Express Inspector will be available to answer any questions you may have.

Outside of London, the hub of the National Express coach network is in Birmingham. The coach station at Digbeth, near to the Bull Ring Shopping Centre, has recently completed a major refurbishment and now offers a new restaurant, toilet facilities for the disabled and additional information points. The end of 1990 will also see the start on major improvements to Victoria Coach Station in Central London making it even easier for coach travellers arriving or departing from the Capital.

THERE'S MORE TO NATIONAL EXPRESS

National Express can offer the coach traveller a lot more than just a coach service from A to B.

A range of Bargain Breakaway Short Break holiday packages can be arranged to around 60 destinations throughout England, Scotland and Wales.

A Bargain Breakaway holiday package gives you the flexibility to decide not only where you want to go but also how long you want to stay, which coach to take to get there and what to do once you have arrived. Accommodation ranges from top quality hotels to small family run guest houses, all offering exceptional value for money. Prices include your accommodation and return coach travel from your nearest National Express or Caledonian Express pick-up point.

The Bargain Breakaway brochure also contains details of London Theatre Breaks offering a weekend (or longer) in London, theatre tickets for your chosen show, return coach travel and a free Travelcard for use on London's central bus and Underground network.

AIRPORT TRAVEL MADE EASY

The recently improved network of coach services linking most parts of the UK with all the major airports has seen a continued increase in the number of people taking the coach and leaving the car at home. Even so, with many flights scheduled for departure early in the morning or arriving late at night, it is sometimes necessary to start travelling at an unfavourable time of the day. To avoid this, National Express and Caledonian Express have a range of Airport Stopover breaks which combine the advantages of coach travel with a hotel situated near to the airport. Taking an Airport Stopover break means that you can travel down to the airport hotel the night before, have a good night's sleep and check-in the following morning feeling refreshed and ready to enjoy your holiday. Coming home and arriving at the airport late at night, you can check in to your Airport Stopover hotel leaving the final part of your journey until the next day.

INTO EUROPE WITH NATIONAL EXPRESS

Taking the coach to the rest of Europe may not have even entered your mind, yet more and more people are discovering that popping over to Paris or Amsterdam by coach is a great way to discover these continental destinations.

The network of European coach services is called Eurolines and offers scheduled express services to around 190 destinations stretching from Finland to Portugal and from Poland to Italy. Eurolines coaches leave from London's Victoria Coach Station and will normally stay with you through to your destination.

It is worth remembering that the distances involved can be quite high and, although regular stops are made along the route, packing some sandwiches, a good book and some comfortable shoes can be an excellent idea.

Full details of all Eurolines services can be obtained from any National Express or Caledonian Express agent.

HAVE A GREAT DAY OUT WITH NATIONAL EXPRESS

With around 1500 destinations from which to choose, taking the coach for a great day out gives you the opportunity to discover lots of new and exciting places.

A day's shopping in Chester or London or sightseeing in York or Stratford can make a welcome change with special day return fares, advertised locally, to many popular destinations.

If there's a group of you travelling together you may be able to get a discount on the fare, giving you even more money to spend once you reach your destination.

If you belong to a club or group and are planning an excursion or other group outing, Crusader Group travel will find a suitable coach for you at a price that probably can't be beaten. Details of Crusader Group Travel will be found in the 'phone book.

THANK YOU FOR TRAVELLING WITH US

The aim of all National Express and Caledonian Express staff is to make your journey as enjoyable and as comfortable as possible and to ensure that you reach your destination safely and on time. To find out more about the many services that National Express and Caledonian Express have to offer, you are invited to call in to any one of the 3,000 appointed agents throughout the UK or to telephone your local telephone enquiry centre, the numbers are in the phone book.

Coach travel has improved tremendously over recent years and it is destined to improve even further in the years to come. With such a wide choice of services, a range of low fares that offer excellent value for money and a commitment to service that is second to none, next time you want to travel around the country, here's a very useful hint . . . get together with National Express.